CBD OIL

THE GIFT OF NATURE

International Edition

Dr Peter Baratosy MB BS FACNEM

CBD OIL

THE GIFT OF NATURE

International Edition

Dr Peter Baratosy MB BS FACNEM

Review of previous edition of *CBD Oil: The Gift of Nature.*

I was very fortunate to be able to review Peter's book. It's a wonderful summary of Peter's personal experience with Medicinal Cannabis and Cannabimimetic molecules as well as an in-depth summary of the evidence available to date, of the mechanisms by which CBD can contribute to the management of the myriad of health conditions it can be used for. It's full of both hard science and personal anecdotes, which makes it an especially enjoyable read.

CBD Oil: The Gift of Nature can be used both as a textbook for clinicians, and as a resource for patients who would like to learn more about CBD, PEA, and other holistic health solutions.

Dr Orit Holzman BSc, MB BS PhD
Vice President of the Australian and New Zealand College of Cannabinoid Practitioners (ANZCCP)

I was so excited to read Dr Peter Baratosy's latest book about medicinal CBD and PEA. The informative and well researched book discusses the mechanism of action, and the receptor systems involved, as well as some of the colourful worldwide history of the use of cannabis. Best of all are the presentations and individual patient case studies, which speak of the wonderful applications of CBD oil and PEA and how they safely reduce suffering and restore health. These benefits often have occurred where other treatments have been ineffective or produced unacceptable side effects.

It was also very interesting to read of the legalities associated with the use of CBD oil.

Thanks Peter. Bravo!

Dr Linda Wilson MBBS BMed Sci

This book is written for general information only – is not intended for diagnosis or treatment.

The author, editor and publisher accept no responsibility for any adverse reaction caused by lack of consultation with a qualified doctor or practitioner, including responsibility for any personal decisions made by the reader in relation to his or her or any member of their family's self-diagnosis.

Peter Baratosy Books
Huonville, Tasmania

Printed in Australia
Cover Design: Nikola Boskovski
Editor: Karen Mace
ISBN: 978-0-6451053-2-2

TABLE OF CONTENTS

DEDICATION

Dedicated to Jenny – my better half! Thank you for giving me the idea to write this book and for your ongoing love, support, and encouragement. I could not have achieved this without you.

Part 1
An Introduction to
Cannabidiol Oil

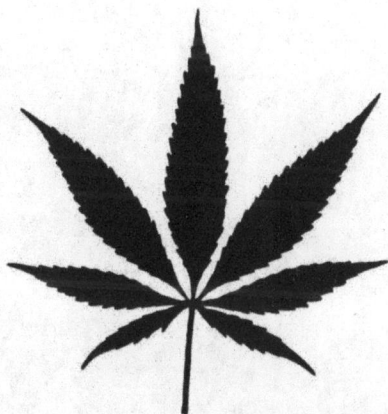

Chapter 1
Introduction and background to use of medicinal cannabis

The study of medicinal cannabis (MC) flowed from my long-time interest in natural medicine. After much study and research, and seeing positive patient responses, the next step seemed to be to share my experiences of the many benefits of this humble plant. This book came about because I wanted as many as possible to know about the many almost magical qualities and great healing power of this plant.

Research shows that the body has a cannabinoid system known as the endocannabinoid system (ECS). This system has been in the human body for millennia and allows the body to make its own cannabinoids. The cannabis plant has a molecule that is similar to what the body makes. This is analogous to the situation with opium. The poppy has a molecule similar to the endorphins that the body produces, hence that plant molecule has an effect on the body.

As I studied and read about the ECS, I realised that there are natural ways of enhancing the ECS. The main cannabinoid of the body is anandamide, which is broken down quickly to arachidonic acid by the enzyme fatty acid amide hydrolase (FAAH). A natural competitive inhibitor of FAAH is palmitoylethanolamide (PEA). PEA is a substance normally produced by the body, as well as a supplement that is easily purchased without a doctor's prescription. This was one nutrient that I could use without going through all the official paperwork required to prescribe MC.

If FAAH is inhibited, anandamide is not metabolised and thus remains available for a lot longer. PEA is not a cannabinoid, but it augments the ECS by enhancing the levels of anandamide. Prior to using MC, I used PEA for all my pain patients, as well as in other conditions where PEA, or more precisely, where enhancing the ECS, would be beneficial. Of course, I continued to use all the other tools I had in my toolbox, such as diet, nutrition, vitamins, minerals, herbs, bio-identical hormones, acupuncture and prolotherapy, as well as conventional pharmaceuticals as needed. The outcomes for all those I treated with PEA showed that PEA worked.

Habib et al. (2019) supported the idea that inhibiting FAAH could be beneficial in treating pain.

This paper describes a 66-year-old woman who presented with no analgesia requirement after a painful hand surgery. Further questioning revealed that she had a lifelong history of painless injuries and burns that healed normally, and she had never needed to take any pain medications. Investigation results showed elevated levels of anandamide and PEA. The researchers also found an abnormal form of the FAAH gene. This all fits together. An abnormally functioning FAAH gene leads to anandamide and PEA not being metabolised, resulting in pain relief for that person.

Many people have a distorted view of the legalisation of cannabis, considering it to be nothing less than a legal way of obtaining cannabis for recreational purposes. In the USA, some states allow cannabis for recreational use; these are the hybrid cannabis plants that contain a high tetrahydrocannabinol (THC) content.

Another aspect of cannabis is the medicinal use. Cannabis has been used for thousands of years as a medicine. I get very annoyed when people refer to cannabis as a drug. I consider cannabis an herb—an exceptionally useful herb. And I consider cannabidiol (CBD) oil an herbal extract.

In this book, I will discuss only the medicinal use of cannabis, and only the CBD component. I will also discuss PEA for reasons I will elaborate on later.

In Australia, there are four standard pathways to access MC:

1. Special Access Scheme (A, B, C): Schedule 5A sub-regulation 12 (1A) item 1 and 1A

2. Authorised Prescriber: Schedule 5A sub-regulation 12 (1A), item 1 and 1A

3. Clinical Trial: Schedule 5A sub-regulation 12 (1A) item 3

4. Schedule 5A contract manufacturing: Schedule 5A sub-regulation 12 (A) item 5

However, there is also a fifth way:

Extemporaneous compounding: Schedule 5 sub-regulation 12 (1) item 6.

This allows compounding pharmacists—those suitably qualified, and licenced with the Therapeutic Goods Administration (TGA), to compound MC, specifically CBD oil, on a regular prescription, issued by any registered medical practitioner for a specific patient, without TGA approval.

Addendum – from the 28 April 2022, this regulation has been amended. Now ALL CBD prescriptions, including Compounded products must have TGA approval.

The Free Dictionary (2020) defines a Compounding Pharmacy as,

"A facility where drugs are compounded or prepared in customised dosages or formulations, typically at the re quest of a physician and for use by an individual patient."

Compounding pharmacists are specialist pharmacists who mix up lotions and potions, capsules, creams, troches, suppositories, and other treatments from raw materials and/or drugs in a form that are generally not manufactured by pharmaceutical companies. They can also make up desiccated thyroid capsules and bio-identical hormone creams.

Compounded CBD oil is classed as a Schedule 4 (S4) item. An S4 is one that requires a doctor's prescription. Compounding pharmacists can also compound CBD/THC products. While TGA approval is not required, state Department of Health approval is, as these products are classed as a Schedule 8 (S8) item. An S8 item is a controlled drug such as opioids and THC, which needs special prescribing authority.

I started prescribing CBD oil and quickly began noticing its benefits. People who, up to that point, had not been helped by conventional means were overcoming many conditions. However, only a short while after starting to prescribe the oil, I discovered that the federal regulation I believed applied to my practice did not apply in Tasmania—they have their own state laws.

Although compounded CBD was an S4 product in the rest of Australia, in Tasmania it was classed as a *poison*, which only specialists could prescribe. To be considered a specialist, you needed Department of Health (DoH) recognition, and to prescribe MC, the specialist had to complete a mountain of paperwork. Tasmania had the most stringent laws regarding CBD in the whole of Australia. The Tasmanian Government had its own cannabis scheme—the Controlled Access Scheme (CAS), which began in 2017.

Under the government's scheme, only relevant specialists could prescribe cannabis (e.g., neurologists, paediatricians, pain specialists) in conjunction with the DoH. One of the main problems was finding a relevant specialist who would be willing to participate. The scheme was very complicated and since its inception, reports Josh Harris (2021), they have approved only nineteen applicants.

There was a seven-step process to achieve this:

1. General practitioner (GP) consultation. If the GP believed that cannabis was indicated, then the GP had to refer to a relevant specialist. (Try finding a specialist who would be willing to assist).

2. Specialist consultation. (Here again, the specialist would have to be willing to assist).

3. Specialist considers cannabis to be appropriate. (Many specialists were unwilling to consider cannabis or are not educated enough to understand its benefits).

4. The specialist applies to the Secretary of the Tasmanian DoH.

5. A delegate of the secretary of the DoH under the Poisons Act, 1971, reviews the application.

6. Delegate issues authority to prescribe to the relevant specialist.

7. The specialist prescribes the cannabis in accordance with the authority, to be dispensed by a Tasmanian Health Service Hospital Pharmacy.

The prescription could only be dispensed through a Tasmanian Health Service Hospital

Pharmacy—generally the Royal Hobart Hospital. The one positive thing was that the state government subsidised the cost of the prescription. Cost is a big factor in MC prescriptions.

Around this time—mid-2020, the Australasian College of Nutritional and Environmental Medicine (ACNEM) sponsored another MC course, a Cannabis Masterclass. Because of the COVID-19 pandemic, states were locked down, face-to-face conferences were cancelled (I had already had to cancel two conferences that I booked earlier in the year), and online meetings became the norm. Optimistic that the laws in Tasmania would change soon, I registered for the class.

On December 3rd, 2020, a historic vote at the United Nations recognised the medicinal value of cannabis and removed it from the list of dangerous drugs. On March 16th, 2021, the Premier of Tasmania, Peter Gutwein, announced changes to the MC laws; from July 1st, 2021, Tasmanian GPs would be allowed to prescribe MC products.

At first, I was sceptical, but then I reasoned that as Mr Gutwein had announced a specific date, from a political point of view, he had to do what he said, otherwise he would be branded untrustworthy. In contrast, if he announced that he would do it "in the future", or "next year", or "soon," then he could probably get away with it if it didn't happen. In the end, Mr Gutwein fulfilled his promise. From July 1st, 2021, Tasmanian GPs could finally prescribe CBD oil without needing to go through the DoH. Doctors could apply to the TGA for approval, or use compounded CBD oil, which does not need TGA approval. However, CBD plus THC prescriptions still need Tasmanian DoH approval to be prescribed. The Tasmanian CAS system is still in place—meaning that the Tasmanian Government will still subsidise the cannabis if the CAS system is used. If the script is done privately through a GP, there will not be any subsidy from the Tasmanian Government.

At this point, I started prescribing CBD again.

Chapter 2

What is CBD Oil?

Medicinal Cannabis as an all-encompassing term refers to any extract from the cannabis plant used for medicinal purposes. This includes CBD oil as well as combined CBD and THC products of various ratios, as well as the individual content of terpenes and flavonoids.

I will *not* discuss THC in this book, mainly for medico-legal reasons — although I will mention it at times for completeness of a discussion.

First, a THC prescription is designated as prescribing an S8 drug which needs special approval from the TGA and the various state Departments of Health. Compounded CBD/THC may not need TGA approval but does still need a state DoH approval. This adds to the bureaucratic complications.

Second, at present, in most states of Australia, the law says that having detectable amounts of THC in your system while driving is an offence prosecutable under law. The law does not differentiate between those who may be under the influence of a recreational drug and those who are taking a medically prescribed substance. The mere presence of THC detected by the road-side test is all that is necessary for prosecution. THC is a fat-soluble molecule and can be detected in the body for weeks after taking a dose.

Towell and Fowler (2020) reported that the Australian state of Victoria was considering changing the law in that state. On October 20th, 2020, just a few days after their article appeared in The Age newspaper, the Victorian Government agreed to change the driving laws regarding MC patients. However, at the time of writing, that law has not yet been implemented, and it remains that, for now, only those taking cannabidiol-only medications can lawfully drive. Once the law is implemented, reports Tom Brown (2021), those using MC, which contains variable amounts of THC, will have the same rights to drive as patients using legal drugs such as opioids.

In Tasmania, the laws are different again. Drivers with detectable THC in their saliva are not prosecuted if they have a valid prescription for the THC. This is most likely because of the Tasmanian Government's CAS, where the state government subsidises MC. However, drivers may still be prosecuted if the police consider the driver to be *driving erratically* or *driving under the influence*.

What is CBD oil and what does CBD stand for?

CBD stands for cannabidiol—a major component of the cannabis plant. There are many components of the plant and, as research continues, more are being discovered. In fact, there is some confusion about how many cannabinoids there are. Lafay, Karila, Blecha and Benyamina (2017) state that there are over 500 components of cannabis, of which 104 have been classified as cannabinoids. Newer figures are higher, indicating that new cannabinoids, albeit minor ones, are constantly being discovered. A quick Internet search brings up many varying, broad figures depending on which website you look at. Some state 104, others, 80-100, and still others, >100. The number continues to grow.

More recent papers, such as that of Cather and Cather (2020), show even higher numbers, mentioning a figure of 113 cannabinoids, while Zagzoog (2020) suggests there are over 120. With more research, this number will possibly increase.

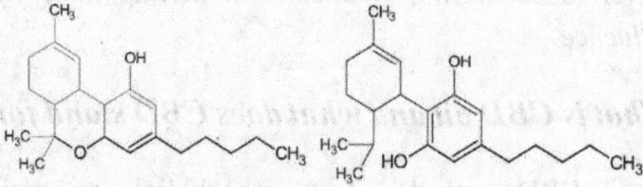

Tetrahydrocannabinol and Cannabidiol

Below are just some of the cannabinoids other than CBD and THC:

CBDA (cannabidiolic acid),

CBN (cannabinol),

CBG (cannabigerol),

CBC (cannabichromene),

CBL (cannabicyclol),

CBV (cannabivarin),

THCV (tetrahydrocannabivarin),

THCP (tetrahydrocannabiphorol),

CBDV (cannabidivarin),

CBCV (cannabichromevarin),

CBGV (cannabigerovarin),

CBGM (cannabigerol monomethyl ether),

CBE (cannabielsoin),

CBT (cannabicitran)… and there are many more.

We are not yet sure of what individual properties all these various cannabinoids have. More research needs to be done. The ones that have been researched the most are CBD and THC. Note that a full spectrum CBD oil can contain some of these other cannabinoids as well as the CBD. A CBD isolate only contains CBD.

Some cannabis plants also contain tetrahydrocannabinolic acid (THCA). It is important to note that it is THCA that is in the cannabis plant, and not THC. THCA needs to be converted, or *decarboxylated* (i.e., the acid component - the carboxyl (COOH) group, is removed), to produce THC; this occurs with heat (smoking, cooking), with light, and with ageing. THCA is not psychoactive, while THC is the main psychoactive component of cannabis.

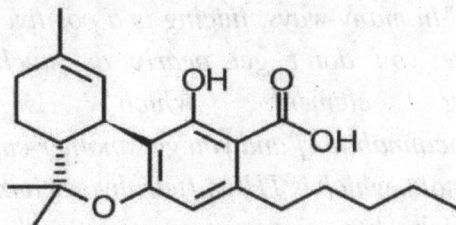

Tetrahydrocannabinolic Acid (THCA)

The following story presented by the ABC (7.30 Report, March 7th, 2018) highlights both the benefits and challenges of using THCA medicinally. A father was treating his sick daughters with cannabis. Both daughters had severe Crohn's disease. Although both were taking many pharmaceutical medications, they were not doing well. In fact, they were dying. The father took matters into his own hands and started treating them with cannabis leaf smoothies. He was using the leaf and stem only and not heating it therefore, there was no psychoactive THC; the leaf contains mainly cannibidiolic acid (CBDA) and THCA. Within weeks, they improved, put on weight, and were getting close to a remission. Police raided him and charged him with cultivation and possession of cannabis. Eventually he was not jailed but put on a good behaviour bond.

In an article referring to the above story, Michael Vincent (2018) quotes Iain McGregor, Professor of Psychopharmacy at the Lambert Initiative for Cannabinoid Therapeutics at Sydney University, "*Juicing cannabis is much different from smoking it.*" He continues, "*In many ways, juicing is a positive thing to do because you don't get nearly as much of the intoxicating element, which is THC [tetrahyrdocannabinol] and you get another component of cannabinoid, which is THCA [tetrahydrocannabinolic acid], which has very strong anti-inflammatory properties in the gut.*"

Heating cannabis in any way including, burning, smoking, and cooking, converts THCA which is not psychoactive into THC which is psychoactive. So, eating cannabis as a salad, or drinking it as a smoothie, has many medicinal benefits without the psychoactive effects.

In the same vein, raw cannabis contains CBDA, which is the parent compound of CBD. CBDA is converted to CBD via decarboxylation when burned, vapourised, heated, dried, stored, or in the process of CBD extraction. This reaction also occurs with time, although slowly.

CBDA has very similar properties to CBD, however CBDA is much more active. Cannabis that is unprocessed, such as raw product made into a smoothie, has a higher content of CBDA than CBD. The acid part of CBDA, i.e., the COOH part, is structurally like many of the non-steroidal anti-inflammatory drugs (NSAIDs) and therefore has anti-inflammatory properties. In fact, the results of a study by Takeda, Misawa, Yamamoto, and Watanabe (2008) showed CBDA is a powerful, specific cyclooxygenase 2 (COX-2) inhibitor.

Note: the initiation and progression of inflammation involves the cyclooxygenase (COX) enzymes.

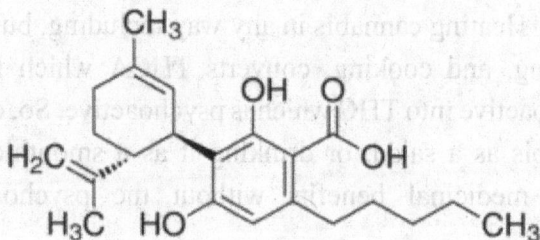

Cannabidiolic Acid (CBDA)

Rock and Palmer (2013) have shown CBDA to be much more potent than CBD in nausea in an animal model. This seems to be because of potent enhancement of 5-HT (serotonin) receptors, according to Bolognini et al. (2013).

CBDA also has been shown to be more potent than CBD in a mouse model of acute inflammation (Rock, Limebeer, & Parker, 2018).

CBDA seems to be absorbed more effectively than CBD and this was demonstrated by Pellesi et al. who published their findings in 2018. The outcome of their study was that THCA and CBDA were absorbed better than THC and CBD.

CBDA downregulates COX-2 in human breast cancer cells, while the basic helix-loop-helix family member E41 (BHLHE41) gene, a suppressor of breast cancer metastasis, is upregulated. Since a major cause of death from breast cancer is metastases, COX-2 downregulation and BHLHE41 upregulation may help reduce metastatic growth (Takeda et al., 2014).

CBDA comes in various products. Special extraction techniques are necessary to extract the CBDA without converting it to CBD. A full spectrum CBD contains some CBDA.

We can go back even further. The mother of all cannabinoids is cannabigerolic acid (CBGA). All cannabinoids start from CBGA, which is then converted by the various plant enzymes (depending on species/hybrid) to CBDA, THCA, cannabichronic acid (CBCA), and the other cannabinoids.

The different strains of cannabis have different ratios of THC (technically THCA) to CBD (technically CBDA); however, the total amount of THCA and CBDA is the same. That is; where there is high THCA, there is low CBDA, and vice versa (Alger, 2013).

A third major component is the terpenes. These are important components of the cannabis extract and therefore are discussed in a dedicated section later.

A fourth component of cannabis is the flavonoids.

***

Flavonoids are a group of polyphenolic substances that are found in most plants, fruits, vegetables, grains, bark, shoots, stems, tea, and wine. These phytonutrients are responsible for the different colours in the plants, fruits, and vegetables. The substances are known for their health-promoting properties (Panche, Diwan, & Chandra, 2016). Over 6,000 flavonoids have been discovered in nature and about twenty have been discovered in cannabis. There have been two flavonoids discovered that are specific to cannabis: Cannflavin A and B (Barratt, Scutt, & Evans, 1986). Both flavonoids have significant anti-inflammatory activity.

Some of the other flavonoids in cannabis include:

Quercetin–which helps relieve allergy symptoms and reduce high blood pressure, also found in apples, berries, brassica vegetables, capers, grapes, onions, shallots, tea, and tomatoes, as well as many seeds, nuts, flowers, barks, and leaves (Li et al., 2016).

Apigenin–which has antioxidant and anti-inflammatory properties as well as blood pressure lowering, antibacterial and antiviral properties, and tumour suppressing effects, also found in chamomile tea, parsley, grapes, apples, red wine, and many Chinese medicinal herbs (Yan, Qi, Li, Zhan, & Shao, 2017).

Kaempferol–which has anti-cancer properties and is also found in apples, tomatoes, grapes, potatoes, onions, and broccoli (Ren et al., 2019), and

Orientin–which is a powerful antioxidant found also in medicinal plants such as *Ocimum sanctum* (Indian holy basil or Tulsi), *Phyllostachys* species (bamboo   leaves), *Passiflora* species, *Trollius* species (Golden Queen), and *Jatropha gossypifolia* (Bellyache Bush) (Lam, Ling, Koph, Wong, & Say, 2016).

So, you can see that the flavonoids also have positive actions on the body in their own right. The combination of the cannabinoids, the terpenes, and the flavonoids all contribute to the entourage effect (Li et al., 2016)

Chapter 3

The Cannabis Plants

Cannabis species belong to the Cannabaceae family. One of the other members of this family is *Humulus lupulus* or hops, used in beer making. The popular opinion is that there are three species of cannabis: *Cannabis indica, Cannabis sativa* and *Cannabis ruderalis.*

Cannabis indica plant originated in the Middle East, in places such as Afghanistan, Pakistan, and Tibet. *Cannabis sativa* is thought to have originated in the warmer areas of Asia and Central and South America. *Cannabis ruderalis,* which originates in Central and Eastern Europe, is very low in THC but high in CBD. The plant itself is shorter than the other species so is not suitable for fibre use, and as it is low in THC, is not used for recreational purposes. However, it does auto-flower, so can be used to hybridise with *sativa or indica.* Auto-flower is where the plant flowers without the need for any special conditions. The two other species need special lighting conditions to flower; it is the flower that contains the most active ingredients. Cannabis is a *photoperiod sensitive* plant, that is, lighting is essential.

Although they still need light to grow buds, cannabis plants begin to flower when they have at least twelve hours of darkness.

Another interesting facet of the cannabis plant is that there are male plants and female plants. The male plant does the pollinating, and the female plant grows the flowers and seeds, which are high in THCA and CBDA. The plant goes through two stages: the vegetative stage and the flowering stage. It will spend the first six weeks or so growing as long and big as possible, and at this stage, goes into *pre-flower* stage. This is when the plants start to show whether they are male or female; the male plants begin to grow pollen sacs, while the female plant grows pistils. The pistils are shown initially by the growth of wispy white hairs, which then form into the buds that form the flower. It is the flower that is sought after. At this point it can get complicated; lighting is crucial unless you have an auto-flower hybrid from *Cannabis ruderalis*. Some plants can even be hermaphrodite–having both male and female parts. This all depends on which plant hybrid you are growing.

There is much speculation and discussion (Sawler et al., 2015) about these two species as separate entities, although over the centuries cross breeding has occurred to such an extent that the distinction between the two has become blurred. There are now many strains, or hybrids, of the cannabis plant, each with its own unique levels of THCA, CBDA, other cannabinoids, terpenes, and flavonoids.

Another cannabis type is hemp, which is a variety of *Cannabis sativa*. It is grown for industrial use, mainly for its fibre content. The fibre is used to make cloth, paper and building products. In the past, hemp was used for rope making, and for sail making, contributing greatly to the *Age of Sail* through the 15th to 19th centuries. In fact, as all the ropes and sails used on Captain Cook's boats were made of hemp, we could say that the hemp plant played an important role in the discovery of Australia! Hemp has a little to nil content of THC, but significant amounts of CBD.

In 1533, King Henry Vlll ordered that every farmer set aside a quarter of an acre for every 60 acres of land for growing hemp. The penalty for not doing this was a fine of three shillings and fourpence. This was done to make more rope, sails, nets, and other naval equipment. The British Navy had to be built up, and they needed hemp for this to happen.

Chapter 4
Cannabis Use Throughout History

Cannabis use did not start with the hippies in the 1960s. It has been present for millennia. Even before the 1533 edict of King Henry VIII for growing of hemp, cannabis use had been around for thousands of years, both as a fibre and as a medicine. Evidence of cannabis being used to make hunting nets by the Gravettians, an Upper Palaeolithic culture, has been dated back to the era 24,980 to 22,870 BCE (BCE–Before Common Era, or Before Christian Era, is the same as BC, Before Christ. In the same vein, CE–Common Era is the same as AD–Anno Domini–the year of Our Lord. Historians are using BCE and CE instead of BC and AD to steer away from religious (Christian) connotations). Evidence from Taiwan shows that cannabis plants were used more than 10,000 years ago as a medicine, fibre crop, a food, and an entheogen. An entheogen is a psychoactive substance that alters perception, mood, thinking and behaviour; shamans and priests used it for religious or magical purposes.

The use of cannabis for medicine can be dated back to the Chinese Emperor *Shen-Nung* 神農, (around 2700 BCE). He is often referred to as the Yan Emperor and is regarded as the *Father of Chinese Medicine*. Some consider him as a mythological ruler, so whether he existed or not is not certain. However, he is reputed to have written the *Shen-Nung Pen-tsao Ching* (神農本草經) also known as *The Classic of Herbal Medicine* or the *Divine Husbandman's Materia Medica*. *Shen-Nung* is alleged to have had a habit of testing herbs on himself to assess the effects and unfortunately, he died from the toxic effects of one of the herbs. He regarded cannabis as a treatment for senility, appetite stimulation, rheumatic pain, constipation, and female disorders.

Another famous Chinese text, *The Yellow Emperor's Classic of Internal Medicine* or *Huang Ti Nei Ching* (黃帝內經) written by The Yellow Emperor, *Huang Ti* (黃帝), (2698 – 2598 BCE), also refers to the use of cannabis as a medicine.

There is more evidence that cannabis was being used in ancient China. In 2018, a tomb of a shaman from about 700 BCE, near Xinjiang province was excavated. Among the artefacts found was a wooden bowl filled with cannabis of high THC content. Here, the psychoactive properties of cannabis become relevant.

The excavation of tombs at the Jirzankal Cemetery found wooden braziers filled with burned stones and traces of high THC cannabis. The cannabis was thought to be used for funerary purposes.

The famous Chinese physician *Hua Tuo* 华陀 (c 140-208 CE) was thought to use cannabis as an anaesthetic, so he could do surgery painlessly.

Cannabis is mentioned in ancient Egyptian texts, the Ebers Papyrus (c 1550 BCE), the Papyrus Ramesseum lll (c 1700 BCE) and the Berlin Papyrus (c 1300 BCE). The texts indicate that cannabis was used as a suppository for haemorrhoids, as a poultice for infections, as a pessary for gynaecological disorders, and for non-specific eye disorders.

Assyrian texts from around 1800 BCE showed that cannabis was used for grief, epilepsy, as a fumigant and as an insecticide. One translation indicates it was used as a "Drug for Sorrow," which possibly could mean that it had been used for depression.

Cannabis is also mentioned in Ayurvedic texts from ancient India. The *Atharvaveda* (अथर्ववेद), from 1000 – 900 BCE, states that cannabis was used for anxiety. The *Sushruta Samhita* (सुश्रुतसंहिता) compiled between 800-300 BCE, recommended cannabis for diarrhoea, catarrh, and phlegm on the chest.

In Persia, a Zoroastrian text, *Zend Avesta,* dated around 600 BCE, refers to cannabis. Cannabis was considered a prohibitive herb as it could cause abortions. Perhaps what was recorded about cannabis and its uses related to the type of plant available, as unlike other ancient texts, which do not specifically mention the psychoactive properties of cannabis, the *Zend Avesta* does, and associates them with evil and dark magic.

The Greek historian Herodotus (c 484-425 BCE) wrote about the use of cannabis by the Scythians, who would enter tents and throw cannabis seeds on hot stones and then *"howl with pleasure"* at the effects!

Greek herbalists, Dioscorides, Galen and Pliny, wrote about the medicinal uses of cannabis. *Dioscorides* (40-90 CE), in his book *De Materia Medica* described cannabis as an anti-inflammatory and anti-oedema herb, and useful in arthritis. The fresh juice, he suggested, was beneficial in earache. His textbook was used throughout the world as a medicinal text for around 1500 years.

An archaeological study carried out in Israel in 1993, showed that cannabis could have been used for labour pain. The remains of a 14-year-old girl with a 40-week-old baby skeleton stuck in her pelvis was found dating to the 4th Century CE. Analysis of grey carbonised material found in her abdominal area showed phytocannabinoid residue. Researchers concluded that the vapours of the cannabis were used to relieve pain of labour and to improve uterine contractions.

There is some evidence that cannabis is mentioned in the Bible. Many bible scholars agree that the words *Kaneh Bosm* - sound similar to cannabis! *Kaneh* meaning reed or stalk, and *Bosm* meaning aromatic could well have been cannabis. This plant was mixed with olive oil to make an ointment, and then used to anoint – even to anoint the sick. CBD oil can be used topically and retains its beneficial properties when used in this way.

Cannabis and its uses spread from China, India, and the Middle East to Europe.

Benedictine nun and author, Hildegard von Bingen (1098 – 1179 CE) encouraged the use of cannabis in Europe. In her book *Physica,* she documented that cannabis is useful for headaches and wound management. She also wrote that a towel made from hemp be used on "sores and wounds". This idea of the healing power of hemp cloth persisted in medieval Europe. A 1480 law for midwives advised, "for Caesarean sections, the mother should be bandaged with *'a plaster made of three eggs, hemp cloth and Armenian earth,'* after the operation."

The *Codex Vindobonensis 93,* a 13th Century Italian copy of an earlier work (this manuscript, named after the ancient Roman name for Vienna, Vindobona, is now held in Vienna), contains an illustration of the cannabis plant (with its distinctive leaves) above an illustration of a bare-breasted woman. The illustration suggests the use of cannabis mixed into an ointment and rubbed on the breasts to reduce pain and swelling.

Nicholas Culpepper (1616-1654) mentioned cannabis in the well-known book, *The English Physitian (Complete Herbal),* written in 1652-1653. What is interesting about Culpepper's reference to the herb, is that it is the use of the root that is mentioned. He recommended it for jaundice, colic, heavy bleeding, dry cough, and burns. The German physician, Georg Eberhard Rumph (also known as Rumphius), (1627-1702), recorded the use of cannabis root for gonorrhoea in 1696. *The New English Dispensatory* (1764 edition) also recommended the use of cannabis root, boiled, to treat gout and skin inflammation.

William Brooke O'Shaughnessy, (1809-1889), an assistant surgeon working in India with the East India Company became interested in the use of cannabis. He saw great therapeutic benefits, including antiemetic, appetite stimulation, muscle relaxation and anticonvulsant properties being achieved with the plant. He introduced hemp to England. Other physicians quickly became interested and cannabis, or, *Indian Hemp,* began to be used. Even Queen Victoria, (1819-1901), is thought to have used cannabis monthly for relieving her menstrual cramps. Her personal physician, Sir J. Russell Reynolds, (1828-1896), wrote in 1890, *"when pure and administered carefully, [cannabis] is one of the most valuable medicines we possess."*

Cannabis products were in an oil base and administered in drop form, not smoked. The use of cannabis grew. It was used for many conditions, including anxiety, depression, insomnia, migraine prophylaxis, dysmenorrhoea, many forms of gynaecological problems and tremor of Parkinson's disease. Many wrote, and published, papers in the *British Medical Journal, The Lancet,* and the *Journal of the American Medical Association,* confirming the properties and benefits of cannabis.

Cannabis continued to be used regularly as a medicine until the mid-1930s when legal restrictions in the USA were imposed. The reasons for this are many, and will not be discussed in detail here, but the banning came soon after the alcohol prohibition era, (1920 to 1933), ended. One reason could have been that the agencies that once dealt with alcohol prohibition no longer had work, and to prevent budget cuts, they used the opportunity to look to some other substance to concern themselves with. Politics also played a big role. While the American public was familiar with cannabis as a medicine, the word *marijuana* was unknown. After the Mexican Revolution, many thousands of Mexicans crossed the border into the USA to escape from the post-revolution chaos and took with them the habit of smoking cannabis, something not in the general American consciousness. Although there are some theories about the origins of the word marijuana, its actual origin is unknown. It was the Mexicans who took it to the United States, and the anti-cannabis factions continued to use the term to drive the anti-Mexican sentiment. Marijuana sounded more exotic, more Mexican, more foreign, than if they used the common name, cannabis.

One theory is that the name came from the Chinese, *ma ren hua* (麻仁花), 'hemp seed flower'.

Since cannabis did not come under any of the existing classifications, it was easier to class it as a narcotic, even though technically it isn't, than to make up a new classification. As such, it came under the jurisdiction of the Federal Bureau of Narcotics. Harry Anslinger (1892-1975), the first director of this Bureau, led an almost fanatical campaign against marijuana. He was convinced marijuana would corrupt the white

American youth. In a testimony to Congress, he said, *"Marijuana is the most violence-causing drug in the history of mankind ... Most marijuana smokers are Negroes, Hispanics, Filipinos, and entertainers. Their satanic music, jazz and swing, result from marijuana usage."* This statement would be quite laughable in today's world.

There was much propaganda that gave the public a very negative view of cannabis. Anslinger used the power of the movie theatre to push his propaganda. One of the most notable movies of this genre was *Reefer Madness* made in 1936. The 1937 Marihuana Tax Act basically banned all hemp products and allowed certain corporations potentially huge profits through promoting synthetic products made from mineral, chemical, petroleum, and fossil fuel deposits that were previously made from natural (hemp) products.

From the mid-30s to relatively recently cannabis was an illegal substance, making use and research next to impossible. Most of the research carried out was done on people using illicit cannabis. Consequently, some of the conclusions reached may be skewed because the use, the dosage, and the quality were not known. Only recently has there been a resurgence in the interest and use of cannabis. It is worth saying that the psychoactive properties of cannabis played a big part in the decision to apply legal restrictions to its use. It is also worth mentioning that, although the CBD component is not psychoactive, it was also included in this prohibition, so the medicinal use of cannabis ceased.

It appears that in ancient times, it was known that some forms of cannabis had psychoactive properties and that other forms did not. Those types that had psychoactive properties were reserved for the priests/shamans for religious or magical purposes, while those that did not were used for medicinal purposes. Of course, they did not know about THC and CBD, but they knew what types to use!

The plant that O'Shaughnessy brought from India was called *Indian hemp*, and as we now know, hemp is low in THC and high in CBD.

It is also important to point out that the information about cannabis is partly assumed, as ancient texts did not call it hemp or cannabis. In some texts, there were illustrations, and the cannabis does have very characteristic leaves. In other texts, the scholars assume it is hemp because they refer to the plant "that can be woven, or spun, or used for rope."

Even in the ancient Chinese texts, the translation of the Chinese characters is assumed, and the exact part of the plant used is not known for sure. The Traditional Chinese character for hemp is "ma" 蔴. (Simplified character 麻). Some have pointed out that if you turn the character upside down, then it looks similar to the cannabis plant and leaf. On the other hand, after the cannabis plant is harvested, it is hung upside down for drying.

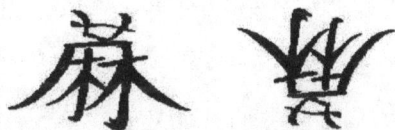

Chinese character for hemp—upside down—looks like a cannabis plant/leaf.

Chapter 5

The Endocannabinoid System (ECS)

Cannabis is one of the oldest medicines known, but why it worked was not understood until recently. While studying why cannabis worked, researchers discovered a whole new regulatory biochemical mechanism. The endocannabinoid system (ECS) has only been known since the 1990s, and there is still a lot to be learned. New discoveries are being made regularly.

In 1964, Gaoni and Mechoulam found that the psychoactive component of cannabis was THC, but this still did not explain how or why it worked. Initially, it was thought that the THC bound randomly to the cellular membranes in the brain, however, later it was found that there are specific sites in the brain to which the THC binds and through which it works—receptors. In 1990, the first cannabis receptor, (CB1), was found and soon after, a second receptor, CB2, was found. These receptors have always been in the human brain and body, even before cannabis was being used or smoked.

Why do we have cannabis receptors?

If there are cannabis receptors in the body it follows that there must be a natural cannabinoid-like substance produced by the body. The body would not make cannabis receptors just in case you may wish to smoke a joint.

Once the CB1 and CB2 were discovered, the search was on for the body's own cannabinoids. The first endocannabinoid (eCB) was discovered by Mechoulam and his lab members, Devane and Hanuš (Devane et al., 1992). They named it *anandamide,* from the Sanskrit word *ananda,* meaning bliss.

The second endocannabinoid, *2-arachidonyl glycerol,* (2AG), was isolated in 1995. Once the cannabinoid receptor and the body's endocannabinoids were discovered, research ramped up as there was a rush to see how it all fitted together.

Further research showed that there is an ECS. The ECS has three components:

1. the endogenous cannabinoids (eCBs)—the two main endocannabinoids are anandamide and 2AG. There are a few other minor ones such as 2-arachidonyl glyceryl ether (2-AGE or noladin ether), N-arachidonoyl dopamine (NADA), and virodhamine,

2. cannabinoid receptors (CB1 and CB2) and,

3. the enzymes for synthesis and degradation of the endocannabinoids. Anandamide or N-arachidonoylethanolamide (AEA) is synthesised in the post-synaptic junction from arachidonic acid, an omega 6 fatty acid. It is mainly broken down by FAAH.

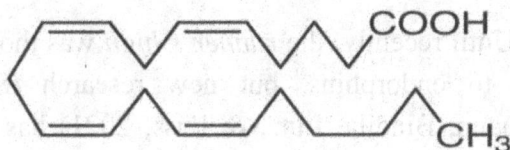

Arachidonic Acid

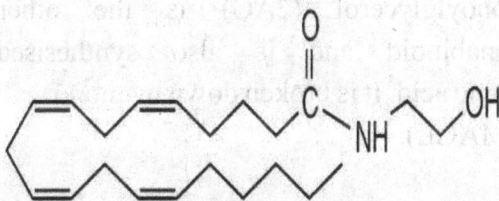

Anandamide

Anandamide has a role in regulating inflammation and in neuronal signalling, as well as regulating feeding behaviour and the generation of motivation and pleasure.

An interesting fact is that paracetamol, also known as acetaminophen, a common analgesic, combines with arachidonic acid via FAAH to form N-arachidonoyl aminophenol (AM404). This metabolite is a weak CB1 and CB2 agonist and inhibits anandamide reuptake; therefore, paracetamol is a pro-drug for a cannabimimetic molecule. This is thought to be the reason for its pain-relieving properties. However, there is the danger of liver toxicity with high doses of paracetamol.

Until recently, the *runner's high* was thought to be due to endorphins, but new research (Siebers, Biedermann, Bindila, Lutz, & Fuss, 2021) has shown this to be due to anandamide.

Exercise does enhance the ECS. 2-arachidonoylglycerol (2AG) is the other main endocannabinoid and is also synthesised from arachidonic acid. It is broken down by monoacylglycerol lipase (MAGL).

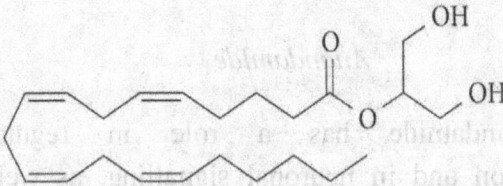

2-Arachidonoylglycerol (2AG)

2AG has been shown to be associated with pain relief, stimulation of appetite, inhibition of vomiting, regulation of the immune system, and inhibition of tumour growth. This endocannabinoid also plays a vital role in the circulatory system, having effects on blood vessels and the heart, and has been shown to be related to the feeling of contentment after orgasm. The results of a 2017 study (Fuss et al.,) showed increased levels of 2AG after masturbation.

The main role of the ECS is to keep the body in a state of homeostasis, that is, to keep the body in balance. When imbalance is detected, the ECS kicks into action; endocannabinoids are synthesised and interact with endocannabinoid receptors that then stimulate a response to return the physiology back to balance. For example, if there is stress, pain, or an injury that throws the body out of balance, the ECS helps return it to normal.

Many of the CB1 receptors are on the nerve synapses, while the endocannabinoids are produced in the post-synaptic area. Unlike neurotransmitters, which are pre-made and stored in vesicles to be released when needed, the endocannabinoids are made by one or two enzymic steps and are released quickly when needed. Basically, the endocannabinoids are retrograde messengers. Technically, the endocannabinoids are made in the post-synaptic area, and the CB1 receptors are in the synaptic area, so when the endocannabinoids are released, they influence the synaptic area and modify neurotransmitter release. This is perhaps the reason why CBD can work very quickly, even in a matter of days, in, for example, anxiety.

eCBs, and cannabinoid receptors have a very important impact on pre- and post-natal development. As we shall see in the section on women's health, anandamide levels are important in conception, implantation, and pregnancy. Post-natal development in the baby relies on eCBs in breast milk.

A high concentration of eCBs is found in mother's breast milk, where the level of 2AG is greater than anandamide (Grant & Cahn, 2005). The eCBs in breast milk are thought to play a role in the baby's learning to latch onto the nipple for sustenance, and they also have a role in stimulating appetite and providing restful sleep. Any interference in this delicate process, such as maternal cannabis use, can cause subtle, but significant, effects on the baby (Fride, 2008).

In a rat model, THC use during pregnancy can alter the development of the offspring's ovaries and have long-term effects on future female reproductive health (Martinez-Pena, Lee, Petrik, Hardy, & Holloway, 2021). At this point, we really do not know if this happens in humans. More research is definitely needed.

However, until further evidence is available, the above are good reasons not to use cannabis while pregnant and, or breastfeeding.

Historically, cannabis has been used for appetite stimulation, so it does make sense that eCBs are in mother's milk. CB1 receptors have a critical role in the motor control of suckling, which also influences energy balance and food intake. Fride, Bregman, and Kirkham (2005), suggest that children with "non-organic ability to thrive," may have a problem with a low ECS tone, or a problem with the eCBs in breast milk, or it could be that they have not been breast fed. Fride (2004) found that anandamide also has a neuroprotective action that helps in the developing post-natal brain.

The information outlined above provides strong evidence for the benefits of breast feeding. However, not everyone can breast feed. If it is not possible, the mother may be able to access a *breast milk bank.* This alternative, however, is still in its early days. If this does become more popular, then storage conditions need to be considered, as they may affect the levels of eCBs and other nutrients (Wu, Gouveira-Figueira, Domellof, Zivkovic, & Nording, 2016).

Chapter 6
The Functions of the ECS

The ECS is a regulatory system that is millions of years old. It coordinates basic biological processes to preserve life. These processes include:

1. Perception of pain and temperature

2. Neuroprotection (brain protection)

3. Heart function

4. Gut function

5. Lung function

6. Cell metabolism—including cellular proliferation and apoptosis

7. Reward and addiction

CB1 receptors are implicated in:

1. Hunger and food intake

59

2. Stress response

3. Reproductive function

4. Sleep cycles.

CB1 is found mainly in the central nervous system (CNS), and to some extent, peripherally, in the endocrine glands, spleen, heart, and some other areas. CB1 is involved in memory, mood, motor function, and pain perception. Of course, CB1 is also related to the psychoactive properties when THC binds to these receptors.

CB2 receptors are involved in:

1. Cellular immune responses

2. Inflammation and wound healing.

CB2 is found mostly in peripheral tissues, especially in the immune system, the gut, and the peripheral nervous system. Cabral, Raborn, Griffin, Dennis, and Marciano-Cabral (2008), discovered that there are some CB2 receptors in the brain, and that these are important for central immune function.

The CB2 receptors found in the immune system are related to inflammation. Therefore, these receptors are involved in conditions such as asthma, allergies, autoimmune diseases, inflammatory bowel disease, rheumatoid arthritis, autoimmune thyroid disease (Hashimoto's and Graves' disease), and other diseases where inflammation is present.

When considering the role CB1 and CB2 play in the human body, as indicated above, it is impossible not to note how useful CBD could be.

Endocannabinoid deficiency

Clinical endocannabinoid deficiency (CECD or CED) is a theory "... *based on the concept that many brain disorders are associated with neurotransmitter deficiencies, affecting acetylcholine in Alzheimer's disease, dopamine in parkinsonian syndromes, serotonin and norepinephrine in depression, and that a comparable deficiency in endocannabinoid levels might be manifest similarly in certain disorders that display predictable clinical features as sequelae of this deficiency.*" (Russo, 2016).

A deficiency of cannabinoids causes many diseases, disorders, and other unhealthy conditions to occur. The term that is used is *ECS tone*. When the ECS tone is low, the ECS needs to be stimulated. Therefore, supplementing cannabinoids could re-balance the system. It is possible to enhance the body's own ECS, or supplement cannabinoids from plants (phytocannabinoids). There is evidence that CECD plays a role in many conditions, especially where conventional medicine has no specific treatment. These conditions include fibromyalgia, chronic pain, anorexia, depression, irritable bowel syndrome (IBS), migraines, multiple sclerosis, post-traumatic stress disorder (PTSD), Huntington's disease, Parkinson's disease, and autism. This list is not exhaustive. The ECS is known to be helpful in reducing inflammation, therefore, any condition where there is inflammation can be treated with CBD oil.

Chapter 7

Palmitoylethanolamide (PEA)

Palmitoylethanolamide (PEA), also known as Palmidrol, is an endogenous (meaning made naturally by the body) fatty acid amide, that has many actions. First discovered in 1957, many studies have shown its usefulness as an anti-inflammatory and analgesic. It is also neuro-protective and shows immune system regulation activity. PEA is not a cannabinoid, although it has been described as a *cannabimimetic*.

When PEA was first isolated, the ECS had not been discovered, so its discovery was an important step forward in understanding how MC works, especially when researchers realised that PEA and the ECS work together. PEA works on many of the receptors that CBD does, and even more.

Di Marzo et al. (2001) demonstrated that PEA has an inhibiting or downregulating effect on FAAH, the enzyme that metabolises anandamide.

Basically, if the enzyme FAAH is inhibited or downregulated, then the anandamide is not broken down as quickly, and it stays around for much longer; therefore, PEA enhances the actions of anandamide. In this way, PEA can produce a cannabinoid type action.

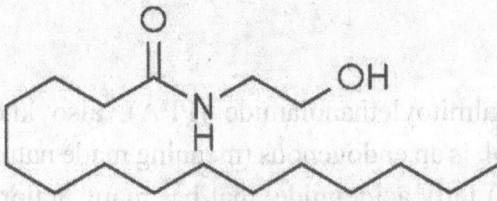

Palmitoylethanolamide (PEA)

***

PEA was shown by Petrosino et al. (2016), to have an affinity to many receptors including Peroxisome proliferator-activated receptor, alpha (PPAR-α), transient receptor potential cation channel subfamily V1 (TRPV1), as well as to cannabinoid-like G-coupled receptors GPR55 and GPR119. PEA is also a cyclooxygenase 2 (COX 2) inhibitor, a microglial inhibitor, a mast cell degranulation modulator, and reduces production of tumour necrosis factor (TNFα) and nerve growth factor (NGF).

PEA does not bind to CB1 or CB2. When PEA binds to the PPAR-α receptor in immune cells, it reduces the production of pain and inflammatory signals such as tumour necrosis factor (TNF) and interleukins.

PEA has been described as a "promiscuous molecule" in that it interacts with many receptors. CBD also does this.

Another way that PEA works is by supporting anandamide as part of the entourage effect. In fact, PEA works on many of the same receptors as CBD. In a response to injury and inflammation, PEA is made locally to deal with the damage, and therefore can be regarded as a self-defence or self-healing molecule (Hesselink, 2013).

PEA is used in many disorders and diseases, including for pain relief, as an anti-inflammatory, in reduction of anxiety, to assist in improving sleep, and to improve mood in depression. It is also helpful in fibromyalgia, peripheral neuropathy, arthritis (pain + inflammation), inflammatory bowel disease, chronic pelvic pain, and vulvodynia. In fact, PEA can be used for many of the same indications as CBD oil.

Although it is quite rare to say that any substance is completely safe, over the more than fifty years of research, evidence has mounted to indicate this *can* be said about PEA. To the time of writing, no interactions, no side effects in short or long-term-use, and no overdose levels have been found. PEA is not addictive, there is no tolerance build up, and there is no evidence of allergic reactions.

***

PEA is made by the body. Why do we need to supplement?

PEA is metabolised by FAAH and N-acylethanolamine acid amide hydrolase (NAAA). Since PEA is broken down quickly, it cannot remain in the body for long in the chronic situation. If the level of PEA is increased, then enzymes cannot degrade the PEA and the anandamide as quickly. In other words, higher supplemented doses of PEA competitively block the FAAH so that the anandamide and the PEA stay around for much longer. PEA appears to be the perfect supplement, but there is one issue.

Oral PEA is metabolised by stomach acid and enzymes. It has a short half-life and a low bioavailability. However, the newer forms of PEA can be micronized, even ultramicronized, to aid absorption. There is now an even more bioavailable form of PEA called Levagen Plus^{TM} (Levagen +^{TM}). This is a clinically studied, superior form of palmitoylethanolamide, that uses a lipid-based drug delivery system, which increases absorption and therefore bioavailability. A study compared 300mg of Levagen Plus^{TM} with 300 mg of normal PEA. The Levagen Plus^{TM} group showed *"increased plasma PEA concentration above baseline concentrations by 1.75 times more than the standard formulation"* indicating better bioavailability (Briskey, Mallard, & Rao, 2020).

PEA is also found in various foods, such as soybean, tomato, corn, milk, egg yolks and peanuts (Petrosino & Di Marzo, 2017). Eating these foods can help with improving health. The benefits of feeding dried egg yolk to underprivileged children living in the poor parts of New York City in 1939 showed that it prevented the recurrence of rheumatic fever, despite the child having recurrent infections with haemolytic streptococcus. Later, children in a convalescent rheumatic home were prescribed four egg yolks daily. No other changes were made with diet or medication. Of the thirty children studied, twenty-four contracted group A strep infections but no recurrence of rheumatic fever. When compared to previous experience, this result was a dramatic improvement. In 1954, a phospholipid fraction was isolated from egg yolk and in 1957, this was shown to be PEA (Hesselink, de Boer, & Witkamp, 2013). Eating eggs can be good for you.

***

The starting dose of standard PEA is 600 mg twice a day. The maximum dose can be as high as 4,800 mg daily. Benefit may not be noted for four to six weeks. For PEA to be effective, it must be taken regularly to build up body levels rather than as needed, as one would with an acute pain medication.

Levagen Plus ™ generally is given at 300 mg twice a day, but the dose can be as high as 2,400 mg a day, and it can be taken for prolonged periods of time.

If PEA is so good and legal, why bother with CBD?

Perhaps one reason is because of the current hype with CBD oil; CBD has gained popularity and is far easier to access now than in the past. My suggestion, as a practitioner, is that if CBD oil cannot be prescribed, then PEA is a good alternative.

A sub-theme in this book is the use of PEA for those who cannot obtain or afford CBD oil. An advantage of PEA is that it is much cheaper than CBD and is now available over the counter at your pharmacy.

PEA works well on its own and can be considered as part of the entourage effect, especially in conjunction with CBD oil. This will be explored in the chapter on the entourage effect.

Chapter 8

Terpenes

Terpenes are aromatic compounds found especially in essential oils, resins, and balsams that produce the characteristic aroma and taste of plants such as lavender, rose and citrus, to name a few.

What does this have to do with CBD?

CBD oil does not contain cannabidiol alone. There are numerous other substances in the plant, including the terpenes, which act synergistically with CBD as well as the THC. Terpenes give the CBD oil, as they do other plants, a characteristic aroma and taste.

The terpenes in the CBD create what is known as the entourage effect. In one study, (Pamplona, da Silva, & Coan, 2018) epileptics were treated either with a CBD-rich cannabis extract or with a purified CBD. The researchers concluded that *"CBD-rich extracts seem to present a better therapeutic profile than purified CBD, at least in this population of patients with refractory epilepsy. The root of this difference is likely due to synergistic effects of CBD with other phytocompounds (entourage effect), but this remains to be confirmed in controlled clinical studies."*

Terpenes include:

Myrcene. Probably the most common terpene in cannabis, myrcene can lower the resistance across the blood-brain barrier as well as having anti-inflammatory and analgesic, antibiotic, and anti-mutagenic properties. The aroma is described as a musky, earthy odour. Myrcene is also found in oil of hops, citrus fruits, bay leaves, eucalyptus, wild thyme, lemon grass and many other plants.

Pinene. Properties include anti-inflammatory, expectorant, bronchodilation, and it is also used as a local antiseptic. As the name implies, this terpene has the aroma of pine.

Limonene. Limonene has been shown to uplift mood and attitude. Also, it has been shown to assist in the absorption of other terpenes. This terpene has a citrus smell like oranges, lemons, and limes.

Beta-caryophyllene (BCP). This is the only terpene known to interact with CB2 receptors. Beta-caryophyllene (BCP) is found in many plants other than cannabis, including Thai basil, cloves, rosemary, cinnamon, and black pepper. The odour is described as peppery, woody and/or spicy.

Linalool. Properties include reducing the anxiety provoking effects of THC. It has been also shown to boost the immune system, reduce lung inflammation and restore cognitive function. Terpene has a flowery and lavender aroma and has calming and relaxing properties.

Terpinolene. This terpene has a CNS depressant action useful in promoting drowsiness and sleep and in anxiety reduction. It is also found in sage and rosemary and has a pine-like odour with slight herbal and floral tones with a sweet citrus flavour.

Camphene. This terpene has been shown, in rat experiments, to affect the cardiovascular system by reducing cholesterol and triglycerides. Camphene has a pungent odour of damp woodlands.

Terpineol. As well as calming and relaxing effects, terpineol has antibiotic and antioxidant effects. The aroma of terpineol is like that of lilacs and flower blossoms and is often found in cannabis strains with high pinene levels.

Phellandrene. It is one of the main compounds found in turmeric leaf oil, and in many other essential oils. Phellandrene is also found in cinnamon, garlic, dill, ginger, and parsley. This terpene has a peppermint aroma.

Carene. While carene has a sweet pungent aroma and is found in many essential oils such as cypress, juniper, and fir needle, it may cause lung irritation when inhaled. This is the reason some hybrids of cannabis with high carene can cause a cough when smoked.

Humulene. This terpene has been found to have anti-tumour, anti-bacterial, anti-inflammatory, and anorectic properties. Humulene is found not only in cannabis but also in hops and Vietnamese coriander.

Pulegone. This is a minor component of cannabis and is also found in rosemary.

Geraniol. This is a terpene that can be an effective mosquito repellent, and medically, has been shown to help neuropathy. This terpene has an aroma like roses.

Chapter 9
The Entourage Effect

The entourage effect is the name given to the mechanism where cannabis components such as THC, CBD, the terpenes, and the flavonoids act synergistically to produce an effect. As mentioned earlier, full spectrum CBD with terpenes and flavonoids works better than CBD on its own. Different hybrids have different terpenes and different flavonoids, and they can have slightly different actions. Some of these terpenes and flavonoids have been shown to have a biological action in their own right. This is like any herb that contains a multitude of different molecules that provide checks and balance actions on the herb.

This is noticeable where pharmaceutical companies extract the *active ingredient*, synthesise that ingredient, and promote it as a drug. When missing all the checks and balances of the whole herb, an isolated active ingredient may not work to the same extent as the herb and/or it may produce unwanted side effects.

In a study of synthetic cannabinoids (SC), Kohen and Weinstein (2018), showed that, *"SC drugs are associated with more undesired effects including agitation, irritability, confusion, hallucinations, delusions, psychosis, and death."* The researchers also posited that there is a correlation between chronic use of SC and a greater risk that a user will develop serious mental health issues than there is when the substance used is cannabis or other psychoactive substances. They concluded that *"SC drugs show greater toxicity than organic cannabis, and therefore further investigation of their long-lasting and acute adverse effects is required as well as better detection and controlling measures against the spread of the use of SC products."*

The whole plant extract is much safer and found to be more beneficial than the synthetic or the purported active-ingredient-only form.

Not all scientists support the idea of an entourage effect, and Cogan (2020) dismisses it as a marketing tool, stating that *"Claims of a cannabis entourage effect invoke ill-defined and unsubstantiated pharmacological activities which are commonly leveraged toward the popularization and sale of ostensible therapeutic products. Overestimation of such claims in the scientific and lay literature has fostered their misrepresentation and abuse by a poorly regulated industry."*

However, other studies (Ferber et al., 2020; Koltai & Namdar, 2020; Russo, 2019) are more positive - terpenes have an effect and work synergistically with CBD.

We know that when compared to a purified extract, the full cannabis extract worked better than a purified extract. That other components act with CBD to cause an entourage effect must therefore have some validity.

The results of a study by Pamplona, da Silva, & Coan (2018) who used purified CBD in some patients and full spectrum CBD (i.e., CBD + Terpenes + flavonoids) in others, in treatment-resistant epilepsy show that the mixture works better than just the pure CBD.

In another study, Blasco-Benito et al. (2018) looked at breast cancer and cannabinoids. The researchers found that a botanical drug preparation, i.e., a full cannabis extract, worked better than just a pure THC.

A full cannabis extract—cannabinoids, terpenes, and flavonoids—has a better action than purified CBD or THC, as they act synergistically with THC and CBD. The purified extract does not work as well. Not known is the mechanism behind this. Santiago, Sachdev, Arnold, McGregor, and Connor (2019) have shown that the terpenes do not work at the CB1 or CB2 receptor level. We need more research to find at what level they do work.

There are many hybrids of cannabis now. The controversy about whether the plant is *Cannabis sativa* or *Cannabis indica* is probably not the main issue. The issue is: what amounts of THC, CBD, and which terpenes and flavonoids are in that strain? Biologists dislike the use of the word strain. Only bacteria and fungi have strains; plants do not. Perhaps hybrid may be a better term.

You may have heard the term *chemovar*. Chemovars refer to the various chemical compositions of the cannabis hybrid; this is based on scientific analysis of the plant. There are three basic types:

Type 1-THC predominant,
Type 2 - equal THC and CBD levels, and
Type 3 - CBD dominant.

Different chemovars also have different levels and contents of the cannabinoids, terpenes, and flavonoids. The only way to know is to have it scientifically tested.

Another word you may hear is cultivar. This is based on what the plant looks like, whether it is short or tall, what shape the leaf is, as well as the smell and physiological effects. What a plant looks like does not necessarily show what the levels of the individual components are; this must be scientifically tested. Therefore, chemovar is a better scientific approach.

Chapter 10
Cannabidiol Oil (CBD Oil)

The more we learn about CBD, the more we realise how complex it is in the way it influences so many receptors and pathways. It is not as simple as initially thought.

It is important to mention that THC does bind to CB1 receptors, hence the prominent psychoactive effects. However, as this book is about CBD, with some discussion about PEA, THC will be mentioned only where it is necessary for clarity.

The eCBs (anandamide and 2AG), bind, as they are designed to do, to both CB1 and CB2. CBD, however, does not bind to either CB1 or CB2.

So how does it work?

It seems that the CBD does not directly trigger CB1 or CB2, rather it modifies the receptors to allow the eCBs, anandamide and 2AG, to bind more easily. In other words, CBD enhances the action of anandamide and 2AG by acting as an *allosteric modulator*. This means that CBD can affect the receptor's ability to function, either increasing or decreasing its sensitivity by changing the shape of the receptor. The CBD does not attach to the active part of the receptor but attaches to the side of the receptor and in doing so, alters the shape of the active part, which modifies its action.

CBD, as mentioned earlier, is considered a *promiscuous molecule,* because as well as interacting with CB1 and CB2, it interacts with many other receptors that enhance the ECS. The same can be said for PEA.

1. Serotonin receptors–CBD can directly and indirectly stimulate the 5-HT1A receptor, which is a subtype of the serotonin receptor, thus producing an anti-anxiety effect. The CBD seems to stimulate the serotonin receptor directly, and it also increases ECS tone to enhance the serotonin receptor indirectly.

2. Vanilloid receptors–one type of Vanilloid receptor is the transient receptor potential cation channel subfamily V (TRPV). The TRPV1 (pronounced as trip V1) receptor has been shown to mediate pain perception, inflammation, and body temperature. CBD binds to TRPV1 and so

does capsaicin, the compound in hot chilli. Capsaicin cream is used to reduce chronic neurologic pain such as postherpetic neuralgia. Anandamide also binds to TRPV1 receptors. All are known to influence pain sensation (Costa, Giagnoni, Franke, Trovato, & Colleoni, 2004).

3. GPR55-CBD blocks this receptor. GPR55 has been shown to cause bone resorption and encourages cancer cell proliferation. Therefore, blocking this receptor produces less bone loss and prevents cancer cell propagation (Whalley, Bazelot, Rosenberg, & Tsien, 2018; Whyte et al., 2009).

4. Peroxisome proliferator-activated receptors (PPARs) - These receptors are in the cell nucleus. Activation of PPARs by CBD, especially PPARγ, produces anti-proliferative effects as well as inducing tumour regression. PPARγ also degrades amyloid plaque and therefore is potentially useful in Alzheimer's disease. CBD can also activate PPARα, which is involved in fatty acid oxidation and is a main regulator of energy homeostasis.

5. Gamma amino butyric acid (GABA) is the main inhibiting (calming down) neurotransmitter in

the CNS. CBD can affect the GABA-A receptor by changing the shape of the receptor, thus intensifying its sensitivity to GABA, and therefore reducing anxiety (Bakas et al., 2017).

CBD also acts as an allosteric modulator at *mu* and *delta* opioid receptors, which are responsible for pain perception (Kathmann, Flau, Redmer, Trankle, & Schlicker, 2006). Hurd et al. 2019 considered this and designed a study to investigate whether CBD's action as an allostatic modulator is why CBD can be used to treat chronic pain, and opioid addiction and withdrawal.

In the various states in the USA where cannabis is legal, there is a lower opioid death rate. The reasons for this are discussed by Bachuber, Saloner, Cunningham, and Barry (2014) who posit the possibility of it being that people are using opioids less, because they can obtain cannabis more easily, or perhaps because cannabis helps to reduce the addiction and, or withdrawal from opioids.

CBD is also an anandamide reuptake and breakdown inhibitor. So, in effect, CBD increases anandamide levels, allowing the body's own eCBs to have a greater effect (Deutsch, 2016).

CBD also alters the shape of the CB1 receptor, reducing the effect of THC. Thus, a balanced THC: CBD product will not produce the same *high* as a THC-only product.

CBD also influences fatty acid binding proteins (FABP), which shuttle eCBs in the cells. CBD and THC can displace eCBs from the FABP and, in effect, enhance the action of the eCBs on the cell surface (Elmes et al., 2015).

Initially, it was thought that CBD inhibited the enzyme that metabolises anandamide, FAAH. However, later research shows that CBD works as a competitive FAAH inhibitor, as FAAH metabolises both anandamide and PEA.

Chapter 11

How to Improve the ECS Naturally

To improve the ECS, it is necessary to understand why the imbalance has occurred in the first place. Following are the most common reasons for imbalance in the ECS.

Stress

Initially, the ECS does its job to balance out the effects of stress. Anandamide and 2AG are increased to help the body cope with the stress. However, if the stress becomes chronic, the continued elevation of 2AG continues to stimulate the CB1 receptor and the brain compensates by reducing or downregulating the CB1 receptors. If there are fewer CB1 receptors, then emotional balance may become more difficult (Morena, Patel, Bains, & Hill, 2016). Stress does affect CB1 signalling. In acute stress, the CB1-ECS signalling is activated to protect the body from the effects of acute stress. In chronic variable stress, the CB1-ECS signalling is reduced, and the resultant deficiency contributes to the negative effects of chronic stress. However, repeated exposure to the same stress can sensitise CB1 signalling, which results in reduced stress response (Hillard, 2014).

Poor Diet

The western diet is high in sugars and unhealthy fats. The ECS controls the appetite, therefore this poor diet produces more eCB in the gut, which increases hunger. Compounding this, fat cells can produce even more eCB, which also increases hunger and makes weight loss more difficult (Donovan, Argueta, & Di Patrizio, 2017; Pagano, Rossato, & Vettor, 2008). Increasing omega-3 fatty acids can help by improving the omega-3 to omega-6 ratio. The western diet has a distorted omega-3 to omega-6 ratio: too much omega-6 and not enough omega-3. Humans evolved with an omega-3 to omega-6 ratio of approximately 1:1. The western diet has an omega-3 to omega-6 ratio in the order of 1:25-1:40. By increasing omega-3 we can balance the ratio. We have seen that anandamide and 2AG are synthesised from arachidonic acid, which is an omega-6 fatty acid. On the reverse side, too much omega-6 can downregulate the CB1 receptors. However, the CB1 receptors need omega-3 fatty acid for their formation. So, a healthy ratio of omega-3 to omega-6 is needed for optimal ECS function. Supplementing omega-3 fatty acids in the form of fish oil, or krill oil and, or, eating a diet with plenty of free-range products can help balance out the ratio. On the other hand, reducing the excess omega-6 can also help. Omega-6 is not bad, it is the ratio to omega-3 that is the issue.

Coincidently, the oil with the best omega-3 to omega-6 ratio is … hemp oil!

Drugs

Mild to moderate alcohol intake has minimal effect on the ECS, but heavy, and binge drinking, can increase the production of eCBs, especially 2AG, and can increase CB1 receptors. However, chronic alcohol intake can over-stimulate the CB1 receptors, and the brain can downregulate these receptors, thus causing tolerance. Long-term alcohol abuse reduces the ECS tone; this change is reversible on abstinence after four to six weeks (Hirvonen et al., 2013). Tobacco smoking can also reduce the density of CB1 receptors in the brain (Hirvonen et al., 2018).

Diseases

Many diseases seem to be related to an unbalanced ECS. This is where the CECD comes into play. We have already touched on this condition. Diseases such as Parkinson's disease, multiple sclerosis, depression, PTSD, glaucoma, arthritis, and schizophrenia seem to be related to an unbalanced ECS.

Those who have these diseases can be helped with CBD, which can balance the unbalanced ECS. Current research supports this theory in migraine, fibromyalgia, IBS, and other treatment-resistant syndromes (Russo, 2016).

Genetics

Here we get into the realm of single nucleotide polymorphisms, or SNPs (referred to as *snips*). With the completion of the Human Genome Project in 2003, many genes were noted to have variations where one or more of the amino acids in the protein chain were different, which led to possible alterations in the function of the protein produced. Proteins are long chains of amino acids, and their function relies on the shape that the chain folds into. Structure, or shape, equals function.

Imagine a string of pearls–they all sit nicely, but if one of the pearls has a different shape, then the whole chain doesn't sit right.

So it is with proteins! Here we must think in 3D.

If the alteration is in a critical position, then the protein folds into a different shape, which then has different properties. A variant amino acid in a non-critical area probably has no, or minimal, effect. This explains the fact that many variants have been found that seem to have no action.

If the protein is an enzyme, then generally there is a reduction in activity (although with some there may be increased activity). If the protein is a receptor, then the receptor would have a different shape and therefore have different properties or sensitivities. These variations, especially if at a critical point, produce altered function.

This information is largely academic because there is no way to test for ECS SNPs in clinical practice. There are various companies that perform genomic testing, but unfortunately, none tests for ECS SNPs.

Earlier, we discussed the case of the lady who feels little or no pain, who, when investigated, was found to have an abnormal FAAH gene. Other researchers (Monteleone et al., 2010) looked at the CB1 gene and the FAAH gene and found SNPs in these genes which they correlated to mood disorders such as bipolar disorder and major depression. In another study, Benyamina, Kebir, Blecha, Reynaud, & Krebs (2011) showed a certain SNP at the CB1 receptor increased vulnerability to addictions. Peiró et al. (2020) found an association between panic disorders and a CB2 receptor SNP.

When researchers Doris, Millar, Idris, & O'Sullivan (2019) looked at SNPs in the ECS, seventy were found in CB1, CB2, FAAH and N-acyl phosphatidylethanolamine phospholipase D (NAPE-

PLD). They also investigated which SNPs influenced obesity, diabetes, and insulin levels. Of the 70 SNPs researched, sixty had no obvious association, but ten did. SNPs are common, and while many do not seem to have any issues, some do. Some of these CB1 SNPs were associated with lower insulin levels, lower body mass index (BMI), and fat mass. The rs324420 FAAH SNP was associated with increased obesity.

Additional research has found more SNPs and associated health problems and diseases. There are many SNPs, and the references below are so you can see which specific SNPs are being discussed. If the disease or condition is related to a SNP, then possibly using CBD or PEA may be an appropriate treatment.

***

ECS SNPs associated with myocardial infarction and plasma cholesterol levels (Chmelikova, Pacal, Spinarova, & Vasku, 2015).

SNP in the CB1 gene associated with alcohol dependence (Marcos et al., 2012).

SNP in the FAAH gene associated with attention deficit hyperactivity disorder (Ahmadalipour et al., 2020).

SNP in CB1 linked to fat distribution in young men. This study (Frost et al., 2010) showed that an SNP in CB1 (specifically rs806381 polymorphism) was associated with fat mass distribution issues, while the rs1049353 polymorphism was not associated.

SNP in CB1 was associated with obesity and metabolic syndrome in postmenopausal Polish women (Milewicz et al., 2011).

SNPs in CB1 and CB2 were associated with depression (Kong et al., 2019).

Another study (Ehlers, Slutske, Lind, & Wilhelmsen, 2007) showed an association between a CB1 SNP and impulsivity in southwest Californian Indians.

A CB1 SNP has been shown to be associated with Tourette's Syndrome (Szejko et al., 2020).

See also Onaivi (2010) and Console-Bram, Marcu, & Abood (2012).

***

As well as supplementing with CBD, there are other ways to improve ECS function. We have already alluded to some:

Reduce Stress: We live is a stressful century, especially now with the COVID-19 pandemic. There are many ways to deal with stress; meditation, yoga, Tai chi, herbs, and exercise are just a few. Change your lifestyle! Change your job! Change your diet! I know … easier said than done.

Exercise: Up until now, the *runner's high* was thought to be due to the endorphin system but is now known to be related to the ECS. Exercise can elevate the blood levels of anandamide and 2AG (Brellenthin, Crombie, Hillard, & Koltyn, 2017).

Sex: As we saw previously, 2AG levels were found to be elevated on masturbation, but this could possibly relate to sexual activity in general. In another study, both anandamide and 2AG were shown to be elevated in sexually aroused women (Klein, Hill, Chang, Hillard, & Gorzalka, 2012).

Diet: The high omega-3 to omega-6 ratio of the western diet can unbalance the ECS, therefore, by eating more fish, or taking more omega-3 fatty acids, and, or, eating less polyunsaturated plant oil, this imbalance could be corrected.

Phytocannabinoids: These are not only found in cannabis, but other plants also have phytocannabinoids, including chocolate, maca, black pepper, nutmeg, kava kava, ginger, and hops. One of the terpenes, beta-caryophyllene (BCP), is found in many plants other than cannabis, including Thai basil, cloves, rosemary, cinnamon, and black pepper. BCP is the only terpene known to interact with CB2 receptors.

Cacao is rich in anandamide, and so are truffles.

Yangonin, one of the six major kavalactones found in kava kava (*Piper methysticum)* has been shown to interact with CB1 receptors (Ligresti, Villana, Allara, Ujvary, & Di Marzo, 2012), hence its use in anxiety, insomnia, restlessness, tension, and pain syndromes.

It can be of great benefit to include foods mentioned above into your diet. Now you can have a good excuse to eat your chocolate–but only the dark chocolate with the high cacao content!

Alcohol and Nicotine: As well as promoting health, reducing alcohol and nicotine can help the ECS.

Sunlight: Fifteen minutes of sun exposure can increase eCBs, especially 2AG (Felton et al., 2017).

Fasting: Fasting can temporarily increase 2AG levels. Perhaps this is the reason behind the positive benefits of intermittent fasting, such as inflammation reduction, heart health, cancer protection, and neuroprotection (Hanuš et al., 2003).

Acupuncture: New research (Hu, Bai, Xiong & Wang, 2017; MacDonald & Chen, 2021; McPartland, Guy, & Di Marzo, 2014), has shown that one way of upregulating the ECS is with acupuncture. Another way of saying this is that acupuncture works through the ECS. In some instances, acupuncture upregulates the ECS, and, in other situations, it can downregulate the ECS (Escosteguy-Neto et al., 2012). Since the ECS is a homeostasis modulator, it must have both upregulating and downregulating functions.

Traditional Chinese Medicine (TCM) practitioners have been using cannabis and acupuncture together for a very long time. This is shown by the writing of Emperor *Shen-Nung* 神農 in 2737 BCE, and Emperor *Huang Ti* (黃帝) (2698–2598 BCE), the Yellow Emperor, in his book the *Nei Ching*.黃帝內經.

Of course, another way to balance the ECS is with the use of CBD oil or PEA–the main topic of this book.

Part 2
Clinical Use of CBD Oil

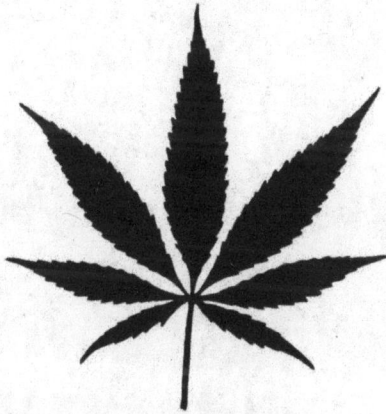

Chapter 12

Introduction to the clinical use of CBD oil

Before I discuss the conditions that CBD is helpful for, I would like to discuss an important point, and that is why doctors are not prescribing CBD as often as, I believe, they should be. This is a question being asked more frequently, particularly given the increasing evidence for its safety and efficacy. My own experience as a prescribing doctor confirms and supports this growing body of evidence.

In a very interesting discussion about physicians' perceptions of medical cannabis, Zolotov, Vulfsons, Zarhin, and Snitman (2018) argue that there are largely two views; those who are negative, who are strongly against its use, and those who are pro MC, who argue strongly for its use. The body of literature addressing this dichotomy grows, and in 2021, Ronne et al. published a systematic literature review of the ongoing discussion. Below I outline the main reasons that doctors do not prescribe CBD.

1. There is nothing about CBD in the medical school curriculum (yet!) and so graduating doctors have no knowledge of its uses or benefits.

2. Fear – fear of using a *natural substance,* fear of using a stigmatised product, and fear of being branded a *quack*! Doctors are very conservative and generally dislike using anything unconventional, although the Royal Australian College of General Practitioners (RACGP) does support the use of MC— at least in principle. A large push for CBD prescribing comes from the people; they research and go to their doctor to request a prescription but are often turned away. Patients then do more research to find a doctor who will prescribe, and if they can't find a doctor who will, then they get it from other sources.

3. The difficulties of completing all the paperwork required to comply with regulations and the legality of prescribing. Most GPs are busy enough as it is; they do not have time to do all the necessary paperwork. I have alluded to this problem already.

4. Despite the significant, and still growing, body of research, many doctors argue that there is not enough. In the following section I will include many references. To the lay reader, I apologise as you may find all these references distracting. To others, the references are included to show that there is plenty of research to

support the use of CBD and PEA. Many of these studies are very recent. Some of these references do refer to animal models of disease but many also refer to the use of CBD in patients. Considering the amount of research already available and the research that is ongoing, I argue that doctors no longer can use the lack of evidence as an excuse for not prescribing CBD.

***

What conditions is CBD oil useful for?

Reiman, Welty, and Solomon (2017), surveyed 2,897 MC patients. The paper lists the reasons for using cannabis. In decreasing numbers - pain (16%), anxiety (13%), back pain, insomnia (9%), migraines, depression (5%), PMT, PTSD, ADD/ADHD, fibromyalgia, inflammation, menstrual pain/cramps, bipolar disorder, muscle spasms, cancer, nausea, loss of libido, diabetes, menopause, Crohn's disease, epilepsy, HIV/AIDS, tinnitus, spasticity, seizures, asthma, and ataxia. Overall, pain, of varying types which includes generalised pain, back pain, fibromyalgia, arthritis, menstrual cramps, was the number one reason, with over 63% of respondents nominating it as the reason for using cannabis.

Although this does not relate directly to CBD oil, the above paper discussed the method of MC usage – 50% of users smoked, 31% vaped and 10% used an edible form. *Note this study was from the USA where MC is supplied as cannabis leaf and flower and not necessarily as CBD oil. As part of the survey, the respondents also said that the MC was just as effective for the pain, with some saying even more so, than opioids, without the dependence, without distressing side effects such as constipation, and without the mental dulling effect.

Another aspect discussed in the Reiman, Welty, and Solomon (2017) paper is the epidemic of opioid deaths in the USA. In just one year - 2016, 63,632 people died of a drug overdose; two thirds of deaths were related to opioids. Scholl et al. (2018) put this into context, noting that there were 58,220 deaths in the whole of the Vietnam war. A substitute for opioids would be very welcome to deal with this epidemic. In places where MC has been implemented, there has been a reduction in levels of opioid use and overdose (Powell, Pacula, & Jacobson, 2018).

There are many diseases and conditions that respond well to CBD oil; however, rather than list them, it is more efficient to categorise conditions into major categories. This classification is based on the lecture of Dr. Philip Blair, who presented in the MC Master Class held in 2020. He arranged the conditions into seven categories. I thank him for his work.

These categories are:

1. Inflammatory
2. Immune
3. Metabolic
4. Neurologic
5. Behavioural
6. Proliferative and
7. Orphan Diseases.

Categorising the conditions gives a fuller appreciation of the benefits of CBD oil. For example, consider inflammation; there are many conditions where inflammation is an issue. Conditions such as arthritis, autoimmune disorders, including rheumatoid arthritis, even metabolic syndrome, which includes diabetes and hypertension, all have inflammation as an underlying issue. Inflammation can also be a trigger for cancer, heart disease and dementia. Dealing with the inflammation can be part of treating all these varied conditions.

Some conditions, however, fit in more than one category. For example, rheumatoid arthritis can be listed under both inflammation and immune categories. Instead of looking at each condition and then looking at lists to see if CBD can help, it is more useful to look at the condition, examine the pathophysiology, and then decide if CBD might help.

Since cannabis has been a restricted item since the 1930s, researchers have had difficulty getting supplies for research. Many of the studies have been done on heavy illicit cannabis smokers, which may give a lopsided view of things. Anecdotal evidence abounds and is readily available on the Internet. While not accepted in the academic world, such evidence can be useful. Then there is the hype. Many companies that make CBD products are biased about their own products.

Much of the information should be considered with a healthy scepticism. I have attempted in this book to refer to published, peer-reviewed studies, not just anecdotes, company biased information, or the hype.

There are several things to consider before accepting the research results as valid and transferable to the world of clinical practice. For example, what product is being used? Do we know exactly what is in the product? Are there contaminants such as heavy metals or pesticides? While there are reputable companies making CBD products, there are also some who are not. US researchers, Bonn-Miller et al. (2018) examined various CBD products purchased online. They found that what was on the label was not necessarily in the bottle. Twenty-six percent of products examined contained less CBD than labelled. Some regulation may be needed to ensure that what you buy—what is on the label—is what you get in the bottle.

You can be reassured that when I prescribe CBD oil, I use a compounded CBD product that is tested for content and purity. The compounded CBD oil contains 100 mg of CBD per millilitre. The reason I use compounded CBD oil is simple – there is virtually no paperwork!

Chapter 13

Inflammatory Conditions

CBD oil can help anywhere there is inflammation.

If you think about it, nearly every disease, every condition, has inflammation as a cause or it at least plays a role in continuing the condition. Therefore, we can treat all conditions with CBD oil, if only to manage any underlying inflammation. CBD oil can deal with inflammation (Burstein, 2015).

PEA also has anti-inflammatory properties. PEA has been shown to be of benefit as an anti-inflammatory generally (Alhouayek & Muccioli, 2014), in neuro-inflammation (Skaper, 2015), in inflammation associated with trauma (Esposito & Cuzzocrea, 2013), in TMJ pain (Marini et al., 2012), and in an acutely inflamed human colon (Couch et al., 2017).

***

Skin

ECS receptors have been found in the skin, so that the skin is considered part of the endocannaboid system. This led to the hypothesis that CBD would be helpful in skin conditions. Karsak et al. (2007) confirmed this by demonstrating that CBD has the potential to alleviate the symptoms of allergic contact dermatitis. More recently, Sheriff, Lin, Dubin, and Khorasani (2020) demonstrated the anti-inflammatory, anti-pruritic, anti-ageing, and anti-malignancy properties of CBD. This confirmed that topical CBD oil or cream can be used with good effect on minor skin conditions such as cuts, ulcers, stings, and burns, as well as on major lesions such as skin ulcers, and other named skin disorders such as eczema and psoriasis.

Some more specific skin conditions also respond well to CBD. Acne, seborrhoea, papules, and pustules were treated successfully with CBD in a study carried out by Ali and Akkhtar (2015). Psoriasis, a common skin disease where there is a hyper proliferation of keratinocytes, responded well to the application of CBD in studies carried out by Derakshan and Kashema (2016), and Norooznezhad (2017). In another, more recent study, Palmieri, Laurino, and Vadala (2019) concluded that CBD is helpful in *"psoriasis... atopic dermatitis and resultant outcome scars."*

The cannabinoid agonist PEA, in a cream form, has been shown to be helpful in treating pruritis (Ständer, Reinhardt, & Luger, 2006). There is no reason why topical CBD would not do the same.

***

Case Study

An 82-year-old lady presented to me with extremely itchy nodules all over the body. Life was miserable as the itching was so intense that she scratched herself to the point of bleeding. She had seen the dermatologist and was diagnosed with Prurigo Nodularis. She had tried a variety of treatments, and none had helped.

When she came to me after being referred by friends, she was taking many medications for diabetes and hypertension. Initially I thought of prescribing CBD oil but because of all her medications, I decided to start PEA 300 mg twice a day. After two weeks she told me that she was much better; the itching had reduced by at least 50 percent. After two months she said the itch was 80 percent better. The skin was healing as she no longer scratched until she bled. I also suggested that she use a liquid form of PEA and apply directly to the itchy areas. She was very happy with the result. She also coincidently mentioned that she was less anxious, her energy levels were better, her diabetes was much better controlled, and she was sleeping better.

***

Musculoskeletal

Problems that CBD may be useful for are muscle joint aches and pains from overuse, trauma, and any form of arthritis. The common treatment for these conditions is the non-steroidal anti-inflammatory drugs (NSAIDs), which, despite being freely available, do present problems with side effects, especially in the elderly. As it is the elderly who most frequently present with chronic pain conditions such as arthritis, they are frequent users. Chronic NSAID use increases the risk for peptic ulcers, acute renal failure, and stroke or heart attack, as well as aggravating heart failure and hypertension. Marcum and Hanlon (2010) stated that NSAIDs caused an estimated 41,000 hospitalisations and 3,300 deaths in the older age category in the year of their study. In another study, Bhala et al. (2013) noted that *all* NSAIDs doubled the risk of heart failure and *all* NSAIDs increased upper gastrointestinal complications.

Anecdotally, CBD is a better choice for pain management as it acts in the same way as NSAIDs, without the side effects. Ibuprofen, a common NSAID, and NSAIDs in general, exert their activity via the *cyclooxygenase* enzymes, (the COX-1 and COX-2 system.) By inhibiting the COX enzymes, the production of prostaglandins, which are involved with inflammation, is reduced. Prostaglandins are made from arachidonic acid and since the eCBs are structurally similar (they are also made from arachidonic acid), this is thought to be the reason CBD has an influence on the inflammatory process (Ruhaak et al., 2011).

While there are some specific COX-2 inhibitor NSAIDs, such as celecoxib, many NSAIDs are a nonspecific inhibitor of the COX-1 and COX-2 enzymes. This leads to side effects despite the NSAID being an effective anti-inflammatory drug. One particular NSAID, ibuprofen, can inhibit FAAH (Deplano et al., 2019), while other NSAIDS can inhibit a possible intracellular transporter of eCBs (Păunescu et al., 2011).The NSAIDs that inhibit COX-2 can influence the ECS because COX-2 is part of the anandamide and 2AG metabolism pathways. CBD reduces the inflammatory response by reducing pro-inflammatory cytokines. CBD seems to be a specific COX-2 inhibitor. COX-1 is mainly expressed in the gastrointestinal tract hence the predominance of gastrointestinal side effects. COX-2 are present at sites of inflammation (Hawkey, 2001).

CBD has been shown to have a relatively good safety profile (Iffland & Grotenhermen, 2017), although longer-term studies are needed. CBD does have some issues which will be discussed later. There is anecdotal evidence that some athletes are turning to CBD oil rather than using NSAIDs. The World Anti-Doping Agency (WADA) in 2018 reversed the ban of CBD products, though THC is still banned (https://www.wada-ama.org › en › questions-answers › cannabinoid accessed 30 Dec 2021). This has led some to switch to CBD products because of their safety profile, and because of the negative side effects of the NSAIDs. A number of studies (Costa et al., 2004; Hammell et al., 2016; Nagarkatti et al., 2009; Russo, 2008; Xiong et al., 2012) have shown that CBD has anti-inflammatory and analgesic properties.

CBD does have an anti-inflammatory effect in rheumatoid arthritis and there is also an antiarthritic effect that is independent of the CB1 and CB2 receptors (Lowin, Schneider, & Pongratz, 2019).

***

Chronic Pain

Although this is one of the most common reasons for CBD use, the question of how effective CBD is in treating chronic pain often arises. Some studies have shown that there are benefits while other studies show minimal effects. Argueta et al. (2020) carried out a systematic review of studies where CBD has been used to treat chronic pain. They concluded, *"In studies of generalized chronic pain, CBD treatment did not significantly reduce measures of pain, however there was consistent improvement in patient-reported quality of life and quality of sleep."*

Despite, according to the results of some studies, CBD not being effective for pain relief, the fact that there are associated benefits, or improvements in anxiety, sleep, and quality of life, indicates that CBD can have a role to play. In contrast, some studies show that CBD does give adequate pain relief to patients and can reduce the use of opioids. *"The results indicate that using the CBD-rich extract enabled our patients to reduce or eliminate opioids with significant improvement in their quality-of-life indices"* (Capano, Weaver, & Burkman, 2020).

The use of topical CBD for arthritis in a study using a rat model showed reduction of inflammation and pain behaviour (Hammell et al., 2016). It should be noted here that as CBD is well known for its anti-inflammatory properties, some of the pain-relieving action could be due to anti-inflammation.

PEA has also been shown to be of benefit in chronic pain of various aetiologies (Gatti et al., 2012), chronic pelvic pain associated with endometriosis (Monte & Marci, 2013), and pain in general (Gabrielsson, Mattsson, & Fowler, 2016). In a double-blind, randomised, placebo-controlled study (Steels et al., 2019), PEA was shown to be beneficial in relief of pain in knee osteoarthritis.

***

Case Study

Mr TS is a 54-year-old gentleman who served in the Royal Australian Air Force (RAAF) and was medically discharged after injuring his back. He suffers from chronic low back pain, anxiety, and PTSD. He also had developed a gambling addiction, mostly as a way of dealing with the chronic anxiety. He was treated with Panadeine Forte tablets (codeine 30 mg with paracetamol 500 mg) and Endone tablets (oxycodone 5 mg), but these were ceased when he developed tolerance and terrible constipation. I started him on CBD oil, and he responded very well.

A report from the pain specialist supported the CBD use and conceded that the CBD had been very effective. A report from his psychiatrist was also very positive. The anxiety, PTSD and irritability were significantly reduced, and sleep greatly improved. He also reduced the Quetiapine from 300 mg at night to 200 mg with the possibility of further reduction in the future. Mr TS also revealed that his addiction to gambling had waned.

***

Infection

No matter whether the cause is bacterial, viral, or parasitic, infection has a degree of inflammation. In the current COVID 19 pandemic, one of the causes of death is the *cytokine storm*. This occurs when cytokines that raise immune activity become too abundant so that immune cells spread beyond infected body parts and begin attacking healthy tissues. The onslaught of these cells can cause leaky blood vessels, fluid retention and a rapid drop in blood pressure. Blood clots form throughout the body, further blocking blood flow so that organs not getting enough blood go into shock leading to permanent damage and even death. Results of a study by Khodadi et al. (2020) demonstrate that the anti-inflammatory properties of CBD oil can reduce and or modify the cytokine storm.

According to Esposito et al. (2020) and Anil et al. (2021), CBD could be useful in treating covid by reducing lung inflammation. In a recent study Nguyen et al. (2021) demonstrated that CBD can inhibit SARS-CoV-2 replication as well as promoting the host innate immune response. This paper is still in the pre-print stage and has not yet been peer-reviewed. PEA has also been suggested as a treatment, or an adjunct treatment, for COVID 19 (Noce et al., 2021; Pesce et al., 2020; Roncati, Lusenti, Pellati, & Corsi; 2021).

Although only demonstrated in an in vitro (test tube) study, CBD has been shown to have the potential to be useful in hepatitis C infections (Lowe, Toyang, & McLaughlin, 2017). And, while the research is yet in its infancy, there are early promising results that CBD may help in some viral infections such as shingles, However, this is more than likely due to the CBD anti-inflammation activity. Mabou et al. (2020) suggest this effect may be more for the chronic after-effects rather than the acute infection.

Antibiotic resistance is a big problem in today's world. CBD has been shown to be a helper compound especially in Gram-positive bacterial infections. According to the research (Wassmann, Højrup, & Klitgaard, 2020) the combination of CBD and antibiotics may be a novel treatment in antibiotic resistant infections.

Initially, it was thought that CBD is not effective against Gram-negative bacteria, but new research (Blaskovich et al., 2021) has shown that CBD was able to destroy a range of Gram-negative bacteria, including *Neisseria gonorrhoeae*, which causes gonorrhoea* and *Neisseria meningitides*, which is responsible for meningitis. This new study also showed CBD benefit against more Gram-positive bacteria such as methicillin-resistant *Staphylococcus aureus* (MRSA) as well as *Streptococcus pneumoniae* and *Clostridium* *difficile*. The authors found that CBD also has *"excellent activity against biofilms, little propensity to induce resistance, and topical in vivo efficacy."*

*In 1696, the German physician, *Georg Eberhard Rumph* (also known as *Rumphius*) (1627-1702) recorded cannabis root as a treatment for gonorrhoea!

**

What about PEA?

The use of PEA in SARS CoV2 has been discussed above. What about other viral infections? Early studies (Bachur, Masek, Melmon, & Udenfrien,1965) have shown that PEA is a non-specific booster of host defences in bacterial and viral infections, as well as a powerful anti-inflammatory.

PEA has been shown to be effective in cold and 'flu and other respiratory virus infections, without side effects. In the 1970s, a Czechoslovakian manufacturer released a PEA product for use in treating colds and 'flus. In this period the results of five double-blind, placebo-controlled studies were published in two separate papers (Kahlick et al., 1979; Plesnik et al., 1977). The group taking PEA had a significant reduction in the development of colds and 'flu compared to the placebo group. Hesselink, Boer, and Witkamp (2013), in discussing the studies carried out during the 70s, commented, *"Taken together, in the period between 1972 and 1977, in total 3627 patients and volunteers completed six different placebo-controlled double-blind trials of which 1937 received PEA up to 1800 mg/day. Relevant side effects were not reported and especially the trials conducted during the flu season demonstrated a treatment, as well as a prophylactic effect."*

Where there is infection, in addition to CBD or PEA, it is beneficial to combine nutrients such as zinc, vitamin D and vitamin C, especially intravenous vitamin C (Huang, Wang, Tan, Liu, & Ni, 2021)) to help deal with infections.

***

The use of CBD in inflammation of various organ.

Lungs. In asthma, chronic obstructive pulmonary disease (COPD) and fibrosis, there is an element of inflammation. In an animal model study, Vuolo et al. (2015) demonstrated the effectiveness of CBD in treating asthma. So far, we have seen that CBD oil can be used orally as well as topically. In asthma, CBD can be vaped or even used in a nebuliser. Another suggestion is to put the CBD oil into a hot cup of tea and sip, which gives the added benefit of inhaling the steam!

Heart. Inflammation is part of the underlying cause of heart disease. In atherosclerosis and hypertension there is a degree of endothelial dysfunction, which has a basis of inflammation and is an underlying cause of heart disease. In a study, CBD was shown to be beneficial in high glucose-induced endothelial cell inflammatory response (Rajesh et al., 2007).

In another study (Abuhassira et al., 2021) older adults who had hypertension were recruited from various hospital departments and were treated with various combinations of CBD and THC. The three-month follow-up of the mean 24-hour systolic and diastolic pressures were reduced by 5.0 mm Hg and 4.5 mm Hg respectively. There were no changes in blood tests, ECG, or anthropometric measurements, indicating that the cannabis was safe

Although CBD does have anti-hypertensive actions this does not necessarily mean that you can stop your anti-hypertensive medication if you start CBD oil. In the long run the hypertension may improve so that the dose could be reduced. When working with any patient, a wholistic approach is warranted, that is, medications are used in combination with diet, weight loss, exercise, nutrients, herbs, and other elements that may be helpful.

CBD seems to have a more underlying benefit to the heart. CBD can reduce the heart response to anxiety or stress, reduce ventricular ectopic beats, reduce the effects of endothelial dysfunction and, limit the size of infarction if CBD is given prior to artery ligation in experimental animals. Again, this is a more general immune systemic effect rather than a direct effect (Stanley, Hind, & O'Sullivan, 2013).

PEA reduces blood pressure in spontaneous hypertensive rats (Raso et al., 2015). But are the results of experiments on rats transferable to humans? Possibly. Even so, I suggest that if PEA is used to treat hypertension, any medication should not be stopped suddenly, rather it should be gradually reduced if, and as, the hypertension improves.

Liver. CBD can help reduce the effects of fatty liver, alcoholic or non-alcoholic type. Fatty liver predisposes to inflammation, cirrhosis, and fibrosis. The ECS is involved in the development of fatty liver (Adejumo, 2017; Alswat, 2013).

Gut. Both CBD and PEA have been shown to reduce inflammation and therefore permeability in the human colon (Couch et al., 2017; Couch et al., 2019). It has been demonstrated that CBD can help reduce inflammation in IBS, inflammatory bowel disease, or Crohn's disease (Schicho & Storr, 2014).

IBS has been considered an example of CECD (Russo, 2008). IBS is a common condition that causes much misery and contributes a huge burden to the health care system. The ECS plays a potential role in IBS and CBD may play a significant role in treating this condition. CBD can be used in situations where there is constipation, diarrhoea, or both. The ECS is a body regulator and so CBD can help to balance the body (Pandey, 2020).

Kidneys. Here again, where there is disease there is inflammation. Autoimmune kidney disease such as IgA nephropathy (Berger's disease) and related glomerulonephritis have a background of inflammation, therefore CBD can help, although it may be an adjunct treatment rather than the main treatment. Using CBD may be a lot safer than using pharmaceuticals to relieve the symptoms. Although the topic has not been fully researched, the use of CBD can help with symptoms of kidney disease such as nausea, vomiting, sleep issues, loss of appetite, muscle cramps and pain.

As mentioned above, PEA can also play a role in protecting the kidneys; in a rat study, PEA protected the kidneys from hypertensive injury in spontaneous hypertensive rats (Raso et al., 2015).

Chapter 14

Immune Conditions

To some extent, immune conditions have been discussed above. Earlier I mentioned that some diseases can be included under more than one category. Autoimmune diseases such as rheumatoid arthritis, systemic lupus erythematosus, multiple sclerosis, scleroderma, Hashimoto's disease, Grave's disease—in fact all autoimmune diseases have an underlying inflammation. CBD can help to manage that inflammation by treating the symptoms such as pain and nausea. Although CBD may not necessarily treat the actual disease itself, it can be a part of the treatment. The same with PEA. PEA has been shown to have anti-inflammatory properties and can be a part of any autoimmune disease treatment (Artukoglu, 2017).

Allergies are another form of immune system dysregulation. While research in this field of CBD use is in its infancy, there is no reason to believe CBD cannot treat allergies. As seen previously, topical CBD can help skin allergies such as eczema and pruritis but what about other allergies?

One of the main contributors to allergies is the mast cells. When these cells are stimulated by an antigen, various factors are released including cytokines, eicosanoids and secretory granules which contain histamine. Histamine is one of the main modulators of the allergic reaction. And as allergies also involve inflammation, the conventional treatments are antihistamines and steroids.

CB1 and CB2 receptors are found on the mast cells and research shows that activating the cannabinoid receptor inhibits mast cell activation and degranulation. This means that *"peripheral cannabinoid CB2 receptors control, upon agonist binding, mast cell activation and therefore inflammation"* (Facci et al., 1995). So, can CBD oil be used for allergies, hay fever, food allergies, asthma, and other allergic reactions?

We have seen that CBD can reduce inflammation, and we have also seen that there are CB1 and CB2 receptors on the mast cells. Thus, as the ECS has control over mast cell activation, there is no reason, theoretically, that CBD cannot help allergies of various sorts.

In a guinea-pig model of asthma, CBD reduced airways contraction of bronchial smooth muscle on antigen exposure (Dudášová et al., 2013).

While anecdotal evidence abounds about the benefits of CBD in treating allergies, there are very few clinical studies to support the many stories of how people have benefited from the use of CBD and its use continues to be controversial. *"Different studies have convincingly demonstrated that cannabinoids play a role in allergy, but their actual contribution is still controversial"* (Angelina, Pérez-Diego, López-Abente, & Palomares, 2020).

PEA also has a controlling action on the mast cells and therefore may be useful in acute and chronic allergies, particularly as PEA is known to be very effective in treating inflammation (De Filippis et al., 2013).

In a case study of the use of PEA in autism, other than just looking at the autism symptoms, the researchers found coincidently that the allergic symptoms also reduced *"nose-picking, asthmatic cough, allergy stigmata (dark circles under eyes and nasal itching), nasal oedema, and both skin eczema and urticaria diminished clinically after a month of PEA administration"* (Antonucci, Cirillo, & Siniscalco, 2015). If PEA works for allergic type issues in autism, there is no reason this outcome cannot be generalised to other populations.

PEA also targets NGF. Many studies have shown that NGF is a key molecule. It not only has an action in nervous system physiology, but NGF is now considered to be an important factor in the pathogenesis of allergic disease. PEA does influence NGF, which in turn impacts on mast cell degranulation (De Filippis et al., 2013; Kytikova et al., 2019).

PEA has also been shown to reduce itch and inflammation in a mouse model of contact allergic dermatitis (Vaia et al., 2016).

CBD and PEA may not cure allergies and hay fever but may be a safe treatment to try if all else fails. Here again the CBD can be put into a hot cup of tea, and you can sip the tea as well as inhale the steam through the nose. This may help with the rhinitis, hay fever and sinusitis.

Chapter 15

Metabolic Conditions

Metabolic syndrome, a cluster of conditions that occur together, is included in this category: type 2 diabetes, hypertension and heart disease, obesity and hypercholesterolaemia. Another facet of metabolic syndrome is the fatty liver, a condition we have already discussed, that CBD can help with. A survey of cannabis users showed a protective effect on non-alcoholic fatty liver disease (Kim et al., 2017).

CBD may not be a cure, but it certainly can be part of the treatment, as underlying inflammation appears to be the basic mechanism in the pathophysiology of insulin resistance and metabolic syndrome (Esposito & Giuliana, 2004; Reddy et al., 2019; Welty, Alfaddagh, & Elajami, 2016).

The use of anti-inflammatory medication has been shown to have a modest effect of treating metabolic syndrome (Esser, Paquot, & Scheen, 2015). The use of CBD as an anti-inflammatory can be part of the treatment. CBD on its own may not be sufficient but other approaches such as weight loss, diet, nutrients, herbs, and medications need to be used. CBD can also help with weight loss and liver protection.

A study by Waterreus et al. (2016) who looked at metabolic syndrome in people with a psychotic illness (who seem to have a high incidence of metabolic syndrome) showed benefit among those who used cannabis. About a third of those studied had used cannabis in the past year. In those who were frequent users and occasional users, unadjusted analysis showed that there were significantly lower odds of developing metabolic syndrome. In the adjusted analysis, the association remained unchanged with frequent users, but the association was lost with occasional users. Cannabis, particularly the CBD component, seems to have a protective effect on the development of metabolic syndrome.

Another way CBD can regulate metabolism is by stimulating the mitochondria, the energy producing organelles that are found in every cell in the body. This has ramifications for all sorts of diseases and conditions. CB1 receptors have been found in the mitochondria outer membranes which makes it likely that CBD can act on the mitochondria. Calcium seems to be the key regulator of mitochondrial energy production (Griffiths & Rutter, 2009), and CBD targets mitochondria to regulate the calcium metabolism (Ryan et al., 2009). It appears that CBD primes the mitochondria to improve energy production and therefore can improve body functioning.

CBD in conjunction with tetrahydrocannabivarin (THCV), one of the other components of the cannabis plant, showed benefit in glycaemic control in type 2 diabetes (Jadoon et al., 2016). CBD may not cure diabetes, but it can make control easier and may help to prevent complications, especially when used in conjunction with diet, exercise, herbs, nutrients, and other helpful elements of wellness.

The ECS is a regulatory mechanism. One of the functions is to regulate food intake. In general, CB1 receptors increase food intake; THC which stimulates the CB1 is known to cause the *munchies*, however, according to Rossi et al. (2018) *"Stimulation of CB2 limits inflammation and promotes anti-obesity effects by reducing food intake and weight gain."* These findings support those of Parry and Yun (2016) who concluded that *"... the current data suggest that CBD plays dual modulatory roles in the form of inducing the brown-like phenotype as well as promoting lipid metabolism. Thus, CBD may be explored as a potentially promising therapeutic agent for the prevention of obesity."*

Interestingly, in their discussion of results of a recently completed study, Spanagle, and Bilbao (2021) suggested that appetite decrease due to CBD was a negative side effect. However, in many cases appetite decrease may be a positive thing.

CBD does not necessarily reduce cholesterol levels but can improve mitochondrial energy function and therefore improve cholesterol transport which can improve cardiovascular health.

As PEA has been shown to reduce inflammation, it therefore would be useful in treating the underlying inflammation in metabolic syndrome. PEA can also be of benefit in the treatment of diabetic complications such as peripheral neuropathy (Schifilliti et al., 2014).

There is considerable evidence that the use of CBD and PEA in metabolic syndrome is beneficial. It can be a positive adjunct to other modalities such as diet, nutritional supplements, exercise, and herbs in the treatment of type 2 diabetes, heart disease, obesity, hypercholesterolaemia and fatty liver. Medication may also be used. These can be reduced (deprescribing) if, and when, there is improvement.

Chapter 16
Neurologic Conditions

This category includes conditions such as headache, migraine, pain in general, Parkinson's disease, Huntington's disease, Alzheimer's disease, any forms of degenerative neurological diseases, and epilepsy. Glaucoma and tinnitus can also be included in this category.

In the introduction to this section, the results of the cited study (Reiman, Welty, & Solomon, 2017) showed that the number one use of cannabis was for pain relief. While I have already discussed, briefly, the varying opinions about the effectiveness of CBD for pain, in this chapter I make further observations about its use, primarily in the context of neurologic conditions.

One review (Stockings et al., 2018) concluded that cannabinoids are not that effective in chronic non-cancerous pain. While another, earlier review (Boychuk, Goddard, Mauro, & Orellana, 2015), showed that the use of cannabinoids in the management of chronic non-malignant neuropathic pain *"may provide effective analgesia in conditions that are refractory to other treatments."*

Another review of cannabinoids (dronabinol, a synthetic THC preparation; nabilone, also a synthetic THC preparation and nabiximols, a plant extract of THC and CBD) in the treatment of neuropathic pain reported *"... a significant, but clinically small reduction in mean numerical rating scale pain scores (0-10),"* but further commented that the cannibinoids were *"also associated with improvements in quality of life and sleep with no major adverse effect"* (Meng et al., 2017).

Historical documents and current research (Baron, 2018) provide evidence that CBD can help in the treatment of pain and that would also include headaches and migraines. CBD, plus or minus THC, works synergistically with the terpenes and flavonoids to deal with pain. The CECD hypothesis, which implies a low eCB tone, is why people suffer migraines and headaches and the reason why cannabis can be a useful treatment (Leimuranta, Khiroug, & Giniatullin 2018).

Is the CECD hypothesis valid? Possibly. However, its validity is based on the fact that the condition responds to CBD, and this could be considered a circular argument.

Other studies (Sarchielli et al., 2007) have shown a reduced level of anandamide in the cerebrospinal fluid (CSF) of chronic migraine sufferers, indicating a breakdown in the ECS. Although there may not be enough evidence from trials to indicate that CBD can and should be used in migraines and headaches, there is plenty of anecdotal evidence, and preliminary results as well as reasonable neurobiological mechanisms to suggest it is a valid option in treatment, and should at least be tried (Lochte, Beletsky, Samuel, & Grant, 2017). And, of course, further research is needed.

Chronic pain, including headaches and migraines, is the most common reason for the use of cannabis. High THC with low CBD hybrids, especially with high terpenes, β caryophyllene and β myrcene, seem to be the most popular (Baron, Lucas, Eades, & Hogue, 2018; Baron 2018).

There is no reason to suspect that a high CBD with the high terpenes may not be effective as well.

CBD is a safe treatment. Other pain medications such as opioids can be addictive and have too many side effects.

***

What about PEA?

PEA has been shown to have a beneficial effect in migraine with aura when used in addition to the NSAID being used (Chirchiglia et al., 2018). The conclusion was that PEA was effective and safe. Another study (Papetti et al., 2020) carried out in a paediatric population, concluded that PEA, administered for three months, reduced pain severity, and reduced the number of attacks.

The authors of many study reports comment that government restriction of cannabis products limits their ability to satisfactorily conduct research. Another issue that influences the outcomes of studies is that many of those taking part in the studies use cannabis purchased over the Internet or from other unregulated sources, or they are cannabis smokers rather than CBD users. When there is no guarantee of the quality and dose of unregulated products, this, of course, influences the results of any research study.

There have not been any longitudinal, adequate studies of CBD and pain. However, anecdotally, many are using CBD oil, both orally and topically, for pain relief. The other major benefit is that CBD oil is non-addictive, and the safety profile is excellent compared to opioids. If we look to history, there are many ancient writers who make mention of the pain-relieving benefits of cannabis.

We discussed mitochondria in the previous section. CBD has been shown to regulate intracellular calcium levels which can achieve neuroprotection. Neurodegenerative diseases such as Huntington's disease and Friedreich's ataxia have been linked to mitochondrial malfunction and may benefit from CBD (Ryan et al., 2009). Mitochondrial CB1 receptors regulate the energy production in neurones (Bénard et al., 2012) and CBD has been shown to be of benefit in neurodegenerative diseases in general (Fernández-Ruiz et al., 2013).

Parkinson's disease (PD) is another disease that responds well to CBD use (Hortes et al., 2014; Peres et al; 2018). Other studies demonstrated that CBD has a positive effect on non-motor PD symptoms (Crippa et al., 2019), PD psychosis (Zuardi et al., 2009), and PD symptoms of rapid eye movement, sleep behaviour disorder, daily activities, and stigmata (Chagas et al., 2014).

In the Chagas et al. (2014) study, the study numbers were small, and the treatment was for only up to six weeks, but the researchers reported *"significant therapeutic effects."* CBD may not cure PD *per se*, but it *can* treat the symptoms such as spasms, tremor, anxiety, and insomnia which can be quite distressing and make life miserable for these people.

PEA can also be helpful in PD. In one study, Brotini, Schievano, and Guidi (2017) looked at using PEA as an adjuvant treatment for PD. PEA was added to the standard treatment with levodopa. The addition of PEA slowed down disease progression and disability without any side effects.

It is possible that PEA alone, without levodopa, would do the same, although more research is necessary to confirm this. In an animal model of PD, (PD-like changes after treatment with 1-methyl-4-phenyl-1,2,3,6-tetrahyropyridine (MPTP)), PEA reversed the changes, even when PEA was given after the MPTP was given (Esposito et al., 2012).

In a mouse model, PEA did prevent parkinsonian phenotypes in aged mice. PEA reduced pro-inflammatory cytokine expression and showed a pro-neurogenic effect in the hippocampus. The conclusion was that this strategy is a *"valid approach to prevent neurodegenerative diseases associated with old age"* (Crupi et al., 2018).

***

Another condition, essential tremor, a neurological disorder that causes involuntary and rhythmic shaking was not helped by a single dose of 300mg of cannabidiol (Santos de Alencar et al., 2021). However, a longer course of CBD, in a mouse model, did reduce tremors, and this, according to researchers Carlsen et al. (2021), was due to CBD action on cannabinoid receptors on astrocytes in the ventral horn of the spinal cord. In a more general study of the management and treatment of neurological disorders, CBD showed promise in the treatment of anxiety, chronic pain, trigeminal neuralgia, epilepsy, and essential tremor, as well as psychiatric disorders (Fiani et al., 2020). In an older study of movement disorders, Peres at al. (2018) concluded that CBD *"emerges as a promising compound to treat and prevent them (i.e., movement disorders)."*

***

Case Study

Mr PH, aged 85, had been diagnosed with essential tremor many years earlier and his condition was slowly worsening. The tremor was so bad that he could not do very much at all. He had to rely on his wife to do everything for him. He had tried all treatments but either they did not help, and/or the side effects made him worse. He and his wife came to see me with the view of trying CBD oil. He started the CBD oil, and when I reviewed him three weeks later, his wife told me that there was a great deal of improvement. She said the tremor was still there, although she noticed that it had lessened when he was at rest. The biggest improvement was in his moods, his demeanour, and that he had basically re-joined society! He was now having conversations with her and had spontaneously joined in with housework, even drying the dishes without being asked. He was out in the garden and no longer just sat, uncommunicative, inside. Before, his moods were very volatile, and now his moods were stable and pleasant. These results were after only three weeks treatment. He was, at this review, taking 0.8 ml of CBD oil (100 mg/ml). We await further improvement.

***

In a simulated public speaking test, CBD was shown to reduce anxiety and tremors in people with PD. A 300 mg dose of CBD given to PD patients reduced tremor amplitude and anxiety in an anxiogenic situation (de Faria et al., 2020).

Tourette's syndrome is another condition that is characterised by multiple spasms, tics, including blinking, coughing, throat clearing, sniffing, facial movements and vocal tics. This condition has been associated with a CB1 SNP and has been shown to respond to CBD (Jakubovski & Müller-Vahl, 2017; Thaler et al., 2019).

Other than PD, there are many other neurodegenerative diseases where there is a paucity of treatment and where PEA and CBD may provide some benefit. Some, but not all, of these are, Alzheimer's disease (AD), multiple sclerosis (MS), Huntington's disease, amyotrophic lateral sclerosis (Lou Gehrig's disease), spinocerebellar ataxia, and spinal muscular atrophy.

A review of twenty-two studies with a focus on Huntington's disease showed strong evidence for significant improvement with neurological symptoms of spasms, tremors, spasticity, chorea and quality of sleep with CBD (Akinyemi, Randhawa, Longoria, & Zeine, 2020).

Progressive supranuclear palsy is a severe debilitating disease also related to other neurodegenerative diseases. In a case study (Hounie & Vasques, 2019), CBD was shown to improve a patient with this disease.

It seems that, while not able to cure, CBD can be useful in all these chronic neurodegenerative diseases, especially where there really are no beneficial conventional treatments. It shows great promise in the studies carried out so far.

> **CBD and PEA can help to treat the symptoms, not necessarily the disease itself.**

CBD can help in many ways. It reduces brain inflammation, provides antioxidant support, offers neuroprotection, reduces anxiety, may relieve depression, and may help with muscle control and muscle spasms. As mentioned previously, CBD may not be a cure, but it can relieve the symptoms, therefore reducing progression.

***

146

CBD activates PPARγ which has been shown to reduce amyloid in AD (Scuderi, Steardo, & Esposito, 2014). The results of one study (Kim et al., 2019) suggested that the CBD component of cannabis, as an anti-inflammatory and antioxidant, could suppress the main causal factors of AD. However, the researchers also suggested that a CBD/THC mix may be more useful.

The use of PEA in Alzheimer's Disease

There is evidence that PEA can help with AD. In a mouse model, ultramicronised PEA helped to retain learning and memory partly by reducing beta amyloid formation, reducing phosphorylation of tau protein, promoting neuronal survival, and restraining neuroinflammation (Scuderi et al., 2018). In another study (Beggiato, Tomasini,& Ferraro, 2019), PEA was shown to improve AD in an animal model.

Unfortunately, there are no large-scale human studies yet, although there has been a small-scale study (Assogna et al., 2020) of PEA + luteolin (luteolin is a plant flavonoid) in nineteen patients with frontotemporal dementia (FTD). All patients did show some improvement in behavioural disturbances and improvement in frontal lobe functions.

PEA is an extremely safe product so there is no reason not to try it.

Prof. Dale Bredesen, in his book *The End of Alzheimer's* likens AD to a roof with many holes. There is not one thing that you can do to block up all the holes but there are many things you can do to address each of the holes such as diet, nutrients, supplements, hormones, removal of toxins and heavy metals, and reduce inflammation. CBD can be a part of this protocol.

There are virtually no effective conventional treatments for neurodegenerative diseases such as AD. Some of the associated symptoms of AD include anxiety and insomnia and for these the conventional treatment would be some pharmaceutical such as a benzodiazepine. These drugs do have significant side effects and can be addictive. I think that CBD or PEA may be worth trialling, mainly because there is evidence it does help, and because of its safety profile.

***

Case Study

Mrs JH, a 72-year-old, presented with loss of short-term memory. She had seen a physician and was diagnosed with early AD. She and her husband came to me with a copy of Professor Dale Bredesen's book, *The End of Alzheimer's*, and wanted to follow his protocol. It was fortunate that I had also read that book. Not long before this I attended a conference where I met Professor Bredesen who was one of the main speakers. The pre-treatment work-up consisted of blood tests as recommended in the book, as well as checking levels of hormones, homocysteine, and B12. An additional test, since there was a family history—her mother had possible AD—was her APO E genotype. The results showed an APO E 3 / 4 genotype that is suspicious of AD. Her homocysteine was high normal and serum homeostatic model assessment for insulin resistance (HOMA) was in an insulin resistant category, but her B12 was normal. She had low hormone levels— consistent with age. I started with various supplements, initiated some dietary changes, and commenced her on progesterone cream. I showed her husband how to do the Montreal Cognitive Assessment (MoCA) test to monitor her cognitive decline. Later, I started her on CBD oil. She reported that she felt a lot better on the CBD, calmer and much happier in herself, and her mood had improved. Her husband confirmed this. The MoCA test showed that she was stable, with perhaps some improvement. She started with a MoCA score of 23 and improved to 25.

***

The MoCA test, developed by Dr Ziad Nasreddine, is used widely, internationally, and involves a series of thirty questions and tasks which are scored to assess cognitive impairment. It assesses not only short-term memory, but also visuospatial abilities, executive functions, attention, concentration and working memory as well as language and orientation to time and place. Just by the way, in 2018, the then president, Donald Trump made the news when he boasted that he "aced" the MoCA test, scoring 30 out of 30! A score above 26 is considered normal. A score of 18-25 is an indication of mild cognitive impairment, a score of 10-17 is considered moderate cognitive impairment, and a score less than ten is considered severe cognitive impairment.

***

Rare diseases such as Dravet syndrome, an autosomal dominant genetic disease, which causes severe prolonged epileptic fits and most often begins before one year of age, and Lennox-Gastaut syndrome (LGS), a severe form of childhood epilepsy, are both difficult to treat with conventional medications. MC can be added to existing pharmaceuticals to control the seizures. A TGA and Food and Drug Administration (FDA) approved product, *Epidiolex*, which is basically a CBD extract (100 mg CBD per ml), is used in the treatment of these conditions. The addition of the *Epidiolex* does bring relief but generally high doses are needed. There is a safety issue here, the necessarily high doses of CBD can suppress the cytochrome P450 liver enzymes, which inhibits the metabolism of the pharmaceuticals that these children are on and can develop into toxicity. Levels must be monitored. (Refer to the chapter on safety).

CBD can also be used for epilepsy and generalised seizures other than Dravet syndrome (Jones et al., 2010). In an animal model of epilepsy, CBD was shown to be a well-tolerated and effective antiseizure agent (Hriday et al., 2019). The possible reason for this is that TRPV receptors regulate the electrical activity of the brain (Iannotti et al., 2014). CBD does work on many different receptors as already mentioned. Gray and Whalley (2020) posit that three receptors are considered important in epilepsy: TRPV1, GPR55 and the equilibrative nucleoside transporter (ENT1). However, more clinical research is always needed.

Many are considering CBD to treat epilepsy because it is natural, safe, and has minimal side effects. As with other diseases and disorders, medical advice and supervision are essential, as it is not advisable to abruptly stop prescribed medication and to go on to CBD.

PEA has been shown to attenuate epileptic seizures in animal models (Aghaei et al., 2015; Lambert, Vandevoorde, Diependale, Govaerts, & Robert, 2001; Post et al., 2018; Sheerin, Zhang, Saucier, & Corcoran, 2004), but there is minimal research in humans.

***

Glaucoma is a disease of the eye where the intra-ocular pressure (IOP) is elevated. This can damage the optic nerve and the retina, leading to blindness. Smoking cannabis had been shown to reduce IOP but the effect is short lived (3-4 hours), and only produced sustained IOP reduction if cannabis was smoked regularly, which obviously is not sustainable (Tomida, Pertwee, & Azuara-Blanco, 2004). One study showed that a dose of 5 mg THC given sublingually did reduce the IOP temporarily, while a 20 mg dose of CBD did not change IOP, and a higher dose of CBD (40 mg) produced a transient IOP increase. So, to treat glaucoma, a THC/CBD mix is needed (Tomida et al., 2006).

PEA has also been shown to be of benefit in glaucoma. PEA reduced IOP in a series of studies (Gagliano et al., 2011; Rossi et al., 2020; Strobbe, Cellini, & Campos, 2013). PEA was well tolerated and there were no side effects. The PEA also showed higher quality of life scores.

Tinnitus has been considered as a form of sensory epilepsy. Anti-epileptics have been tried but with minimal success (Hoekstra, Rynja, van Zanten, & Rovers, 2011). As CBD has anti-epileptic properties (Silvestro et al., 2019) and CB1 receptors and 2AG have been found in the cochlear nucleus, it follows that CBD may help tinnitus (Smith & Zheng, 2016).

Theoretically, CBD can help tinnitus. There are anecdotes of where CBD has helped, but caution needs to be taken as there is a study, albeit in an animal model, where CBD made tinnitus worse (Zheng, Reid, & Smith, 2015).

In a very recent study, Perin (2020) concluded that "*EC (*endocannabinoid*) modulation of neuroinflammatory responses in the auditory system, in particular by CBD, which is neuroprotective, is anti-inflammatory, undergoes clinical trial as an anxiolytic, and acts on pathways involved in cochlear damage protection, may represent a novel pharmacological approach to hearing loss and tinnitus, although more data are necessary (especially on humans) to assess the therapeutic value of this or other EC* drugs."

CBD and PEA may help with the stress, anxiety and insomnia associated with tinnitus. It is important, however, to monitor, and focus on, the level of tinnitus.

Chapter 17

Behavioural Conditions

In this category we will explore anxiety, depression, insomnia, bipolar disorder, PTSD, obsessive compulsive disorder (OCD), autism spectrum disorders (ASD), schizophrenia and anorexia nervosa (AN).

Evidence continues to mount for the beneficial effect of CBD on anxiety. Below I outline how and why CBD is so effective.

We have seen that CBD influences the serotonin receptor, producing an anti-anxiety effect. CBD also has anandamide reuptake and breakdown properties, and inhibits FAAH, the anandamide breakdown enzyme, thus enhancing the ECS.

CBD is an allosteric modulator, and as such has a modulating action on various receptors. With some receptors CBD can be positive, meaning it makes receptors more sensitive, and with other receptors CBD can be negative, making receptors less sensitive. CBD has a positive modulating effect on the GABA-A receptor, making it more sensitive to GABA, which is an inhibitory neurotransmitter. Basically, GABA inhibits or calms down the brain.

The ECS has been shown to be the main link between external and internal stimuli and the resultant neurophysiological and behavioural outcomes such as fear reaction, anxiety, and stress coping. This allows the organism to adapt to the changing external environment and allows long-term viability, homeostasis, and stress resilience. Any change in eCB signalling can lead to psychiatric disorders. (Lutz, Marsicano, Maldonado, & Hillard 2015).

The ECS, on activation, is involved in regulating the triggering of the hypothalamic-pituitary-adrenal (HPA) axis. Under normal conditions, endocannabinoids seem to maintain low HPA axis activity. In acute stress situations, the ECS dampens the HPA axis thus protecting the organism from the effects of stress. However, chronic stress can block CB1 receptors to produce an exaggerated cellular and neuroendocrine stress response (Gorzalka & Hill, 2009).

Normally the CB1 receptor is stimulated by the endocannabinoids, anandamide and 2AG. If there is a loss of the CB1 signalling caused by repeated exposure to *variable* stress then this leads to anhedonia, (the inability to feel pleasure in normally pleasurable activities), anxiety and persistence of negative memories. However, repeated exposure to the *same* stress can sensitise CB1 receptors thus dampening the stress response allowing the organism to adapt to the stress (Hillard, 2014). Chronic stress can lead to depression-like symptoms caused by this abnormal interaction between the eCBs and the HPA axis. (Riebe & Wotjak, 2011).

In a study previously discussed, Reiman, Welty, and Solomon (2017) found that the second most common reason for using cannabis is anxiety. CBD can stimulate the CB1 receptor and thus helps with relieving anxiety symptoms. There have been many studies where participants have successfully used CBD to reduce anxiety (Blessing, Steenkamp, Manzanares, & Marmar, 2015; Schier et al., 2012).

Conventional treatment is to prescribe some form of benzodiazepine or a selective serotonin reuptake inhibitor (SSRI); both have their own problems and side effects. Considering its safety and effectiveness in managing anxiety, a trial of CBD is certainly warranted. CBD can also help in panic disorder (Soares & Campos, 2017).

PEA can also play a role in reducing anxiety. PEA is known to inhibit or downregulate FAAH, thus allowing anandamide to have a longer-lasting effect. Any FAAH inhibitor can play a role in the treatment of anxiety disorders (Hill et al., 2013). In a study (Steels et al., 2019) where the researchers specifically looked at the treatment of osteoarthritic knees with PEA, it was noted that there was also a significant reduction in anxiety. However, this could possibly be due to the reduction of pain.

***

Case Study

Ms A suffered from extreme anxiety, as well as interstitial cystitis and restless legs. She could not survive without her medications – including amitriptyline, oxazepam and fluoxetine. She had tried many treatments, both conventional and non-conventional. They kept her under control but did not really give her a good quality of life. She had a chance to go to Japan for a holiday, which she really dreaded. She was not a good passenger! She came to me prior to the flight requesting *"something to get her through the flight."* In the past she had to take diazepam. Once in Japan, still very anxious, she was advised to buy CBD oil, which is an over-the-counter drug in that country. She had never tried CBD, but she did start, and things changed dramatically; her anxiety disappeared, she slept better, and she felt that life was back to *normal*. After returning to Australia the anxiety recurred as she ran out of the CBD oil. I prescribed and once again the anxiety disappeared, and life was good again!

***

Post-traumatic stress disorder. Symptoms include nightmares, flashbacks, heightened reactivity to stimuli, avoidance of situations that can bring back the trauma, anxiety, and depressed mood. Conventional treatment includes psychological treatments such as cognitive behavioural therapy (CBT), trauma-focused psychotherapies, and pharmaceuticals such as SSRIs.

Dr James Lake (2014), writes, *"The limited effectiveness of current approaches provides compelling arguments for effective conventional and complementary interventions aimed at preventing PTSD and treating chronic PTSD."* Complementary and alternative medicine (CAM) is used by more than 50% of PTSD patients, and CBD is often incorporated into the alternative approach.

I have met military veterans who tell me that the only thing that helps their PTSD symptoms is cannabis – generally illicitly sourced. While anecdotally, cannabis clearly does help those who use it, many doctors prefer to know what the science says.

CBD, in addition to routine psychiatric care, was associated with symptom reduction in adults with PTSD and was also seen to benefit a subset of PTSD patients with frequent nightmares (Elms, Shannon, Hughes, & Lewis, 2019). In another study, Bitencourt and Takahashi (2018), using animal models demonstrated that *"CBD can both facilitate the extinction of averse memories and block their reconsolidation, possibly through potentiation of the eCB system."* The researchers also stated that more recent studies have shown this to be true in humans as well.

Children can also develop PTSD. The use of CBD oil in children with PTSD was shown to be safe and to reduce symptoms of anxiety. It was considered useful as an alternative to pharmaceutical medications (Shannon, & Opila-Lehman, 2016).

PEA may also be useful in treating depression and PTSD. When the PPARα was activated by PEA it facilitated fear extinction and fear extinction retention, as well as inducing an anti-depressant and anxiolytic action. Although this was in an animal model, the researchers concluded that activating PPARα with PEA may be useful in depression and PTSD in humans (Locci & Pinna, 2019).

***

Depression. CBD has been shown to have anti-depression activity, albeit in an animal model (Schier et al., 2014; Sales et al., 2019).

In a paper published in 2018, Crippa, Guimarães, Campos, and Zuardi concluded that, *"CBD was shown to have anxiolytic, antipsychotic and neuroprotective properties."* They go on to say that CBD should be considered for *"potential use in epilepsy, substance abuse and dependence, schizophrenia, social phobia, post-traumatic stress, depression, bipolar disorder, sleep disorders and Parkinson's."*

It is commonly understood that depression is associated with low serotonin levels. And, as CBD is an agonist of the serotonin receptor, its use can result in higher levels of serotonin being available (Russo, Burnett, Hall, & Parker, 2005).

PEA can also be useful in depression (Sabelli, Fink, Fawcett, & Tom, 1996). In a study where PEA was used as an adjunct therapy with citalopram (an SSRI anti-depressant) there was a rapid onset of antidepressant effects. This indicates the potential for PEA to be a useful addition to a therapeutic approach for those with major depressive disorder (Ghazizadeh-Hashemi et al., 2018). PEA itself, when used as the only treatment, has also been shown to have an antidepressant action (DeGregorio et al., 2019).

***

Case Study

A young lady presented with symptoms of depression. She commenced taking citalopram, and I did advise her that citalopram could take up to two, maybe even three weeks to have an effect. At the same time, based on the study above, I also suggested she take PEA in conjunction with the citalopram. At her four-week follow-up, she was feeling very much better – the symptoms of depression were gone. She told me that this improvement started three days after she commenced the citalopram and the PEA.

Another study by De Gregorio et al. (2019) supports previous findings, as the researchers concluded that *"PEA has potential antidepressant effects alone or in combinations with other classes of antidepressants."*

***

Insomnia. Getting a good night's sleep is very important for both mental and physical health and wellbeing. Lack of sleep has been linked to many conditions, including diabetes, hypertension, obesity, and other disorders that come under the umbrella term of metabolic syndrome.

There are many reasons for a person not being able to fall asleep. These include pain, stress, anxiety, depression, hot flushes in menopausal women and sleep apnoea, to name a few. Other reasons include uncomfortable beds, noise, caffeine, alcohol, and drugs. For many, the use of sleeping tablets is a first line solution for sleep problems, however, it is preferable to treat the cause of the sleep issue rather than resort immediately to a sleeping tablet. CBD is known to help with pain, anxiety, and depression, and it can cause a calmness, which aids sleep. One of the side effects, or possibly a direct effect, of CBD is drowsiness. A dose of CBD at night can help with sleep.

While it is known that CBD improves sleep, more studies are needed to help us understand why it does so. It could be that CBD improves insomnia *per se* or that it improves sleep because of its anti-anxiety, anti-pain, and anti-stress properties. A study by Walsh et al. (2021) from the University of Western Australia showed that MC has a positive benefit in insomnia. The study was a placebo-controlled, double-blind cross-over study using a cannabinoid extract, ZTL-101 (a product from Zelira Therapeutics – they do not reveal what is in it).

***

Case Study

Miss AB aged 26 presented with extreme anxiety and insomnia. She had tried many natural nutrients and herbs with only limited benefit. She was not at all interested in pharmaceutical therapies. I started her on CBD oil (100 mg/ml), commencing at 0.1 ml daily and slowly increasing. She was to stop when she felt a positive benefit. At her four-week follow-up, she told me her sleep was now normal and her anxiety was much less. She was very happy with the results. Of note, she only needed 0.15 ml of CBD oil.

***

PEA also reduces pain and anxiety and helps with sleep. The activation of CB1 receptors leads to an induction of sleep. Although PEA does not bind to the CB1 receptor, PEA can enhance the action of the ECS so that CB1 receptors are activated, which may lead to sleep (Murillo-Rodrigues, 2008). In a double-blind, randomised, placebo-controlled interventional study, PEA was found to be a potential sleeping aid capable of reducing sleep onset time and improving waking cognition (Rao, Ebelt, Mallard & Briskey, 2021).

PEA was shown to have a positive effect on sleep in patients with carpal tunnel syndrome (CTS) (Evangelista, Cilli, De Vitis, Militerno & Fanfani, 2018). Here again more studies are needed to help us understand just how PEA works, whether it is the effect on sleep, or the reduction of the neuropathic pain in CTS, or both that results in the improved sleep.

***

Obsessive compulsive disorder and anxiety are, to some degree, inter-linked. The latest revision of the Diagnostic and Statistical Manual of Mental Disorders (DSM–5) no longer classifies OCD as an anxiety disorder, however the obsessions, persistent and unwanted thoughts, urges or images that are intrusive and a part of OCD cause distress and anxiety. Therefore, CBD or PEA, which have both been used effectively in the treatment of anxiety could be included in the treatment regime for OCD (Blessing, Steenkamp, Manzanares, & Marmar, 2015).

***

Case Study

When Mrs JM, aged 54, presented for her first consultation she had many painful conditions, including osteoarthritic (L) knee, which was "bone on bone," neck pains, (L) wrist pain, (R) foot pain and a condition called lipoedema, a painful hereditary disorder found mostly in women where fat accumulates in various parts of the body, but especially from the hips to the ankles. This accumulation of fat can cause swelling, bruising, and pain ranging from mild to severe. She wanted to try CBD oil. On follow-up she said that she was feeling better, the pain from the lipoedema felt less uncomfortable, the (R) arthritic foot pain was better, and she was walking about much more freely. She was only taking 0.4 ml twice a day (this is 80 mg per day – a relatively low dose). She also told me that her OCD was much better. She did not reveal to me in the first consultation that she suffered OCD. She would normally mop the floor of her house up to five times a day–even if it was not dirty. Now she sometimes does not even mop once a day–and this was after only four weeks of treatment.

***

Autism spectrum disorders (which includes Asperger's) are always difficult to treat. There are many aspects, but insomnia and anxiety are a major feature. The focus should not be the diagnosis, rather it should be to target the symptoms. CBD, because of its benefits in improving sleep and in reducing anxiety, can be of benefit in the treatment of ASD. There are also other ways CBD can be of benefit. One study showed that children with autism had lower serum levels of anandamide, PEA and OEA (oleoylethanolamide), a monounsaturated analogue of anandamide. It acts independently in the ECS pathway and has PPARα activity. The researchers, Aran et al. (2019), suggest that these levels can be used as a stratification biomarker. They also suggest that these lower levels indicate a lower ECS tone. Therefore, prescribing CBD or PEA would have a beneficial effect in that it would increase serum levels of anandamide.

There is a large body of anecdotal evidence to show that CBD helps in ASD, and this is supported by clinical studies. Although currently such studies are few, the number is growing. A retrospective study of sixty children with ASD and treated with CBD showed a 61% reduction of behavioural outbreaks (Aran et al., 2019). A prospective open-label study looking at the use of CBD 30% with 1.5% THC, showed that there was 49% significant improvement, 31% moderate improvement and 14% showed no improvement. The most common symptoms where improvement was seen were restlessness, rage attacks and agitation (Bar-Lev Schleider et al., 2019).

Another study, an observational study, used a CBD:THC ratio of 75:1. Of the eighteen participants, one did not show any improvement and three dropped out due to adverse effects. However, most patients showed some improvement in more than one of the eight symptom categories evaluated: attention deficit/hyperactivity, behavioural disorders, motor deficits, autonomy deficits, communication and social interaction, cognitive deficits, sleep disorders and seizures. There were very infrequent and mild side effects including sleepiness, mild irritability, diarrhoea, increased appetite, conjunctival hyperaemia, and increased body temperature. The side effects were slight and temporary. The CBD was used in conjunction with other medications in ten cases (Fleury-Teixeira et al., 2019).

In a study of 66 days duration, CBD oil was used in 53 children. The results were, overall, encouraging. Self-injury and rage attacks improved in 67.6% and worsened in 8.8%; hyperactivity symptoms improved in 68.4%, no change in 28.9% and worsened in 2.6%; sleep problems improved in 71.4% and worsened in 4.7%; anxiety improved in 47.1% and worsened in 23.5%. The adverse effects, somnolence and change in appetite, were mild (Barchel et al., 2019).

Aran et al. (2021) found mixed results from a placebo-controlled double-blind study of the use of a cannabis extract with THC in a ratio of 20:1 and a purified CBD with THC at a ratio of 20:1. Noncompliant behaviour and parental stress showed no significant difference. However, measurements of disruptive behaviour and social responsiveness score did show improvement.

PEA has also been shown to have a positive effect on ASD. In a randomised parallel group, double-blind placebo-controlled trial, over a 10-week period, children with autism were treated with risperidone plus placebo and compared with risperidone plus PEA. Risperidone plus PEA showed superior efficacy over risperidone plus placebo (Khalai et al., 2018). PEA on its own showed improvement, albeit in a mouse model of ASD, through PPARα activation, restoration of brain-derived neurotrophic factor (BDNF) signalling, improving mitochondrial function, reducing central and peripheral inflammation, and by modulating gut microbiota composition (Cristiano et al., 2018).

In two published case studies, where PEA was used there was improvement in expressive language, cognition and behaviours (Antonucci, Cirillo, Siniscalco, 2015).

ASDs are complex and there is no cure and no specific medication. Some medications do treat specific symptoms such as sleep, seizures, anxiety, and depression, and in conjunction with physical and behavioural therapies, can help. The choice is whether to use pharmaceuticals that may, or may not work, and which can have significant side effects, or CBD, which although it doesn't work in all cases, is very safe. However, no medication whether it be pharmaceutical or otherwise works in all cases.

The choice of whether to try the safe treatment first, lies with the parents. Some prefer to do so, while others prefer to begin with pharmaceuticals. Some of the above studies used THC but in a very low dosage. THC use in children is fraught with dangers, and my recommendation is that THC generally not be used in children.

***

Schizophrenia. The use of cannabis in schizophrenia is controversial. Conventional thinking is that cannabis can cause schizophrenia. However, there are some things that must be considered when discussing this. Problems may occur where there is a genetic predisposition to schizophrenia as cannabis smoking may trigger the disorder, or if there is heavy cannabis use where the user smokes cannabis that is high in THC, or where the heavy use is in the adolescent age group, as the adolescent brain is not fully developed and is vulnerable (Radhakrishnan, Wilkinson, & D'Souza, 2014). The thinking is that it is the THC, not the CBD that is the issue.

The ECS does appear to have a role to play in schizophrenia which seems to be associated with ECS alterations. Anandamide levels in blood are higher in patients with acute schizophrenia than in controls. Where there is clinical remission, anandamide levels are reduced (De Marchi et al., 2003). Some researchers, however, think that the high anandamide is a compensatory mechanism rather than cause.

Anandamide levels were also elevated in CSF (Davies & Battacharyya, 2019) and inversely related to psychotic symptoms. In a double-blind, randomised study of CBD versus amisulpride (a potent antipsychotic) in acute schizophrenia, both were safe, and both demonstrated significant clinical improvement, but the CBD had demonstrably fewer side effects. CBD elevated the levels of anandamide, which was significantly associated with clinical improvement. The researchers suggest that the inhibition of anandamide, specifically FAAH deactivation contributes to the antipsychotic effects (Leweke et al., 2012).

We have discussed single nucleotide polymorphisms (SNPs or "snips") previously. A SNP in the CB1 receptor seems to have some association with schizophrenia—especially the hebephrenic type. *"Our findings suggest that heavy cannabis use in the context of specific CNR1 genotypes (CB1 receptor SNP) may contribute to greater WM (Brain white matter) volume deficits and cognitive impairment, which could in turn increase schizophrenia risk"* (Ho, Wassink, Ziebell, & Andreasen, 2011). In another study, Ujike and Morita (2004) showed that CB1 receptors are increased in subregions of the prefrontal cortex in schizophrenia.

Increasingly the evidence indicates that CBD can be useful in the treatment of schizophrenia, and Davies and Bhattacharyya (2019) suggest it be considered as treatment for psychosis in schizophrenia.

The use of PEA in schizophrenia

Unfortunately, there is little research, and more is needed regarding the use of PEA in schizophrenia. However, it is worth trying, considering how effective it is in treating inflammation, which, as with various brain conditions, is a part of the clinical picture of schizophrenia.

Pro-inflammatory cytokines are used as communication molecules between the nervous and immune systems. Astrocytes and microglia are essential cells that have an important function in the brain. They can be a source of inflammatory mediators which can cause brain inflammation. Glial cells can also release inflammatory mediators when stimulated by pro-inflammatory signals from mast cell activation. This brain inflammation has a fundamental role in various brain conditions which includes schizophrenia. PEA has been shown to reduce the brain inflammation by inhibiting mast cell activation and reducing inflammation generally (Skaper & Facci, 2012; Skaper, Facci, & Giusti, 2014).

Theoretically PEA can help by reducing inflammation and dampening mast cell activation. Also, we have seen that PEA is safe and, as it does not clash with any pharmaceuticals, it could be used even when

the patient is taking the usual pharmaceuticals prescribed
as treatment for schizophrenia.

***

Anorexia nervosa is a potentially fatal psychiatric disorder where the individual, due to an obsession with becoming increasingly thinner, limits food intake to the point where health is seriously compromised. The individual has a clearly distorted body image, and an unrealistic fear of weight gain that results in self-starvation.

Cannabis, especially THC, is known to increase appetite and to cause "the munchies." Studies have shown minor improvement in AN. In a short study using dronabinol (a synthetic THC preparation) patients were given 2.5 mg dronabinol twice a day for four weeks then placebo for four weeks. The medication was well tolerated and there was some weight gain, *"after four weeks of exposure, it induced a small but significant weight gain in the absence of severe adverse events"* (Andries, Frystyk, Flyvbjerg, & Støving, 2014). In another study a higher dose THC was used and there was no effect as the high dose counteracted the weight gain due to side effects. The researchers concluded that overall there is little research, and more is needed (Rosager, Møller, & Sjögren, 2021).

In a study of 2,436 patients diagnosed with AN, bulimia, and eating disorders not otherwise specified, the researchers found that 97% had greater or equal to one comorbid diagnosis; 94% had unipolar depression, 56% had anxiety disorders and 22% had substance use disorders (Blinder, Cumella, & Sanathara, 2006). As mentioned earlier, it is important to consider the symptoms as much as it is to consider the name of the disease, as CBD and PEA can be used to treat those comorbid diagnoses.

The ECS is known to relate to eating behaviour. There is some evidence that AN is related to a disordered ECS, so the use of CBD is warranted.

SNPs are also relevant to AN. Researchers, Monteleone et al., (2009), stated, *"Present findings show for the first time that the CNR1 1359 G/A SNP and the FAAH cDNA 385C to A SNP are significantly associated to anorexia nervosa and bulimia nervosa and demonstrate a synergistic effect of the two SNPs in anorexia nervosa."* This could be why CBD may work in AN.

Another substance that may also be useful is PEA (Scolnick, 2018). In a rat model of AN, brain ECS tone was altered suggesting that the ECS is involved in AN pathophysiology (Collu et al., 2019). This is confirmed by another study which showed that *"endocannabinoids and endocannabinoid-related compounds are involved in food-related reward and suggest a dysregulation of their physiology in Anorexia."* (Monteleone et al., 2015).

CBD and PEA do seem to help AN by normalising the ECS, possibly because they help to normalise the variant SNP in the ECS. Also, CBD and PEA can help with the anxiety and depression that is generally associated with AN.

Chapter 18
Proliferative Conditions

Here we are looking at things that grow, such as cysts, tumours, and cancer, benign or malignant. We can also consider in this category the treatment of side effects of cancer therapies, such as chemotherapy nausea. Cancer patients are generally stressed, anxious or depressed, in pain, and have sleep issues. CBD has been shown to help in these situations.

While CBD is not generally used in the treatment of cancer, it could be a very useful adjunct treatment. There is research that shows that CBD does have an action on the GPR55 receptor which is associated with bone resorption and with cancer cell proliferation. An activated GPR55 increases bone resorption and increases cancer cell growth (Hu, Ren, Shi., 2011). CBD is a GPR55 antagonist; it blocks the receptor signalling (Tudurí et al., 2017).

Tumour angiogenesis is inhibited by CBD (Blázquez et al., 2003; Casanova et al., 2003; Solinas et al., 2012.) Angiogenesis is a physiological process where new blood vessels are formed. The growth of any tumour is dependent on angiogenesis. As the tumour grows it needs sustenance and this is provided by new blood vessels growing into the tumour. Without angiogenesis the tumour cannot be sustained and could die off. Note here that angiogenesis is also involved in pregnancy. The growing foetus can be considered as a growing tumour; therefore, CBD is not advised during pregnancy.

A literature review that focused on the biological effects of cannabinoids in cancer treatment, identified *in vitro* and *in vivo* studies specifically targeting pancreatic cancer. The reviewers found that CBD may be an effective adjunct in the treatment of pancreatic cancer. However, they do note the lack of clinical studies and the need for these to be undertaken (Sharafi, He, & Nikfarjam, 2019).

CBD may not be the sole treatment for cancer, but it can be part of conventional cancer treatment (Hinz & Ramer, 2019). It is not only the CBD portion, but the flavonoids that can be of benefit. The flavonoid, FBL-03G, a synthetic derivative of Cannflavin B from the cannabis plant, has been shown to have potential to treat pancreatic cancer. This was demonstrated in an *in vitro* scenario as well as in an animal model (Moreau et al., 2019).

A case report of a patient with adenocarcinoma of the lung was published by Sulé-Suso, Watson, van Pittius, and Jegannathen (2019). An 81-year-old gentleman who declined chemotherapy and radiotherapy, self-treated with CBD oil. A CAT scan in December 2016 showed that the lung tumour had increased in size but a follow-up in November 2017 showed near resolution of the mass. The authors of the report state that previous work has shown that CBD may have anticancer properties and may enhance the immune response to cancer. They asserted that the evidence from this case supports the prior evidence given the *"striking response in a patient with lung cancer."*

CBD also reduces tumour growth in several glioma models (Deng & Stella, 2015). Another study showed that CBD induces "programmed cell death (apoptosis)" in breast cancer cells (Shrivastava, Kuzontkoski, Groopman, & Prasad, 2011). In a similar manner, the endogenous cannabinoid, anandamide, has been shown to inhibit human breast cell proliferation *in vitro*; this anti-proliferative action was not due to toxicity or apoptosis (De Petrocellis et al., 1998). If this is the case, then CBD could help in breast cancer treatment, as CBD does enhance the ECS and anandamide levels.

CBD has also been shown to be a potent inhibitor of prostate cancer both *in vitro* and *in vivo*, either given alone, or in conjunction with commonly used prostate cancer drugs (De Petrocellis et al., 2013). In the same issue of the journal, there is a supportive comment, (Parcher, 2013).

Anecdotal evidence suggests that benign growths such as cysts are helped by CBD oil. There are many anecdotes on the Internet about how CBD was used to treat cystic acne, sebaceous cysts, Baker's cysts, and others, but there have been no studies. Even so, considering CBD has been shown to reduce cell proliferation in malignant cells, then possibly it could also reduce growth in benign conditions. As CBD has been shown to be quite safe, it would be worth trying.

PEA has been shown to inhibit the expression of FAAH and enhances the anti-proliferative effect of anandamide on human breast cancer cells (Di Marzo et al., 2001)

CBD and PEA can also be used to treat the symptoms of cancer such as pain, anxiety, depression, and insomnia, as well as the side effects of chemotherapy, such as nausea, neuropathy, and others. It was demonstrated, albeit in animal studies that CBD can regulate nausea and vomiting and anticipatory nausea that often accompany chemotherapy. The authors also comment that current medications are not always that helpful (Parker, Rock, & Limbeer, 2011). This is supported by Rock, Stich, Limbeer and Parker, (2016).

CBD can also protect against unwanted side effects from chemotherapy. The chemotherapy drug, Paclitaxel, can cause neuropathic pain. CBD has been shown to inhibit this. This study also showed that chemotherapy efficacy is not diminished when patients take CBD during treatment (Ward et al., 2014). Another chemotherapeutic drug, Cisplatin, can cause nephrotoxicity (kidney damage). CBD can prevent this (Pan et al., 2009).

There does not seem to be any contraindication for taking CBD during chemotherapy. The CBD can relieve the pain, reduce the anxiety, help with sleep, relieve/reduce/eliminate nausea, and protect the body from chemotherapy side effects.

Chapter 19
Orphan Diseases

These are diseases where there are no current effective treatments. Here again, CBD may not be a cure but can help to alleviate symptoms and improve life and function. Genetic diseases such as trisomy 21 (Down's syndrome), cystic fibrosis and Huntington's disease are among these diseases. Also included could be anything that mainstream medicine has difficulty treating, such as fibromyalgia. Mainstream medicine can use drugs to control or alleviate many conditions but then the side effects often cause more distress to the person. The treatment, in many cases, could be worse than the disease. Many of the symptoms associated with these diseases such as anxiety, insomnia, aggressive behaviour, and pain could be addressed by using CBD or PEA.

Fibromyalgia is *"characterised by widespread chronic pain, fatigue, and depressive episodes without an organic diagnosis, which may be prevalent in up to 10% of the population and carries a significant cost in healthcare utilization, morbidity, a reduced quality of life, and productivity. It is frequently associated with psychiatric comorbidities"* (Berger et al., 2020). The researchers, who carried out a systematic review of studies looking at the use of cannabinoids in the treatment of fibromyalgia, concluded that although there are not many current good studies available, many retrospective studies and patient surveys show good pain relief, sleep improvement and reduction of associated symptoms.

Fibromyalgia is a chronic health condition that affects approximately five to seven percent of the global population (Cameron & Hemingway, 2020). The disorder is characterised by widespread musculoskeletal pain, with the sufferer often having several comorbidities. Fibromyalgia is associated with high levels of inflammation. Response to traditional pain treatments is poor. In the absence of a definitive cure, treatment is best focused on symptom management and improving quality of life. Cameron and Hemingway (2020) reviewed studies carried out between 2015-2019 and concluded that the studies suggest medical cannabis is a safe and effective treatment option for patients with fibromyalgia. Further research is needed.

The cause of fibromyalgia is not known for sure but there seems to be some form of alteration in the central pain pathways. In one study, increased levels of serum substance P and related analogue hemokinin-1 as well as pro-inflammatory cytokines IL-6 and TNF were seen in fibromyalgia patients, compared to controls. The researchers (Theoharides, Tsilioni, & Bawazeer, 2019) hypothesised that thalamic mast cells contribute to the pain and inflammation by releasing these, and other, substances. They concluded that inhibiting mast cells could be used as a novel way of treating fibromyalgia. It was mentioned earlier that CBD and PEA can stabilise mast cells.

MC has been shown to be beneficial in fibromyalgia and has minimal side effects (Sagy, Bar-Lev Schleider, Abu-Shakra, & Novack, 2019). This study used a combined THC/CBD preparation.

PEA also can be of benefit in fibromyalgia. No medications have shown any significant pain reduction or improvement in the quality of life of the fibromyalgia sufferer. In a group of patients with fibromyalgia, the pharmaceutical regime was helping a little before PEA was added. However, after the addition of PEA, there was significant benefit (Schweiger et al., 2019). In a similar, earlier, study, PEA plus pharmaceutical treatment was more effective than just pharmaceutical treatment alone (Del Giorno et al., 2015).

There is no reason not to try just CBD, or PEA, in fibromyalgia, especially from a safety and a minimal side effect point of view.

Another condition that deserves mentioning here is restless legs syndrome. Those who suffer from this have unusual feelings in their legs, although it can happen in other areas like the arms, chest, and head, Itching, crawling, aching, throbbing and sometimes, pins and needles are some of the sensations the sufferer feels, accompanied by a powerful urge to move the legs in the hope it will make the sensations go away. The mainstream treatment is not always satisfactory, but CBD has been shown to help restless legs (Ghoraveb, 2020; Megelin & Ghoravab, 2017).

Dupuytren's contractures are another condition where the only treatment is surgery, although that would only be in the late stages. In the early stages CBD oil can be used topically and can help.

Below, you can see the difference this made for one person. After only one month, the nodules had reduced in size and are no longer tender.

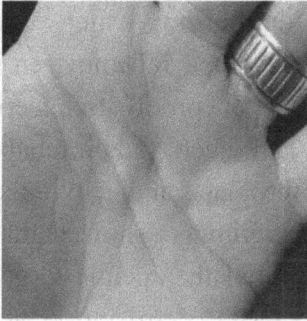

24 October 2020   *22 January 2021*

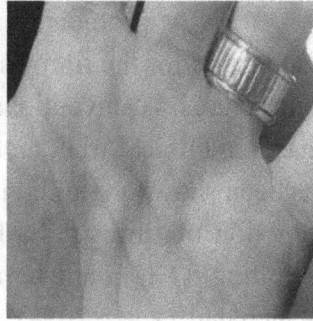

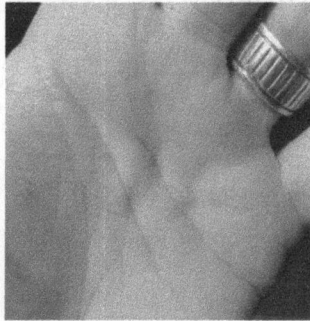

20 March 2021

There is some evidence to support the fact that CBD reduces fibrosis. One study looked at bleomycin-induced scleroderma and used a CBD derivative (VCE-004.8). Bleomycin-induced dermal fibrosis in the mouse model was treated with the CBD derivative. This was shown to reduce the fibrosis by acting on the PPARγ and CB2 receptors (del Río et al., 2016).

TNF promotes myofibroblasts, which are responsible for the fibrosis that develops in Dupuytren's contractures. Conventionally, in a proof-of-concept Phase 2a clinical trial, an anti-TNF agent (adalimubab) has been shown to inhibit myofibroblasts and help in the reduction of fibrosis. Earlier experiments showed that inhibiting TNF could be a potential therapeutic target (Nanchahal et al., 2018). Both CBD (Petrosino et al., 2015) and PEA (Impellizzeri et al., 2015; Hoareau et al., 2009) reduces TNF levels.

Chapter 20
Women's Health

Although not included in Dr Philip Blair's classification of diseases, I felt it important to discuss the clinical uses of CBD in women's health. The ECS regulates almost all levels of female reproduction, and dysregulation of the ECS is associated with development of gynaecological disorders from fertility disorders to cancer (Luschnig & Schicho, 2019). Many gynaecological conditions involve pain, inflammation, anxiety, depression, and insomnia, all of which have been shown to respond to CBD and PEA.

Endometriosis

Symptoms of endometriosis include painful periods (dysmenorrhoea), pain on intercourse (dyspareunia), pain on opening bowels or with urination, heavy menstrual bleeding, bleeding between periods, infertility, fatigue, nausea, constipation, diarrhoea, and bloating. Many of these symptoms can be treated with CBD. One Australian online survey (Armour et al.,

2019) interviewing women from endometriosis support and advocacy groups, found that cannabis, heat, hemp/CBD oil and dietary changes were the most highly rated in terms of reduction of endometriosis pain. In preclinical research, cannabinoid compounds that target the CB1 and CB2 receptors in endometrial tissue appear to control the development of endometriosis (Bilgic et al., 2017). So, while the evidence is good that CBD can help with pain and inflammation and with anxiety and other symptoms, and possibly with the pathological process of endometriosis, there are, at the time of writing, no concluded clinical trials that support this. However, Escudero-Lara et al. (2020) have created a mouse model that mimics some of the conditions of human endometriosis, and using THC, not CBD, they found a reduction in pelvic pain and cognitive impairment. Clinical trials are ongoing to test whether these findings are translatable to patients with endometriosis. There is a study in progress (https://clinicaltrials.gov/ct2/show/NCT045270030) that is looking at the effects of CBD in patients with endometriosis. It is due to conclude in June 2023.

However, there is a study (Stochino Loi et al., 2019) that specifically looked at PEA and endometriosis. The result was that all patients in the study experienced increased quality of life and showed significant improvement in chronic pelvic pain, deep dyspareunia, and dysmenorrhoea. There were no serious side effects.

Historically, cannabis has been used for women's issues. Queen Victoria is reputed to have used Indian hemp for her period pains. Ancient writings showed that hemp/cannabis/CBD was used for *women's problems* in Ancient China and Ancient Egypt.

Menopause

The symptoms of menopause include anxiety, insomnia, aches and pains, mood swings, and osteoporosis, all of which can be helped by CBD and PEA.

The ECS is known to influence the female reproductive system including folliculogenesis, oocyte maturation and ovarian endocrine function. There is a complicated interaction between the ECS and the hypothalamic-pituitary-ovarian axis. Exogenous phytocannabinoids, such as CBD, have been shown to have benefit (Walker, Holloway, & Raha, 2019). CB1 and CB2 receptors are found in the CNS, including the hypothalamus and pituitary gland. Oestrogen has been shown to be involved in the ECS, especially in having a downregulating effect on FAAH; when oestrogen is high, FAAH is downregulated, and therefore anandamide levels are higher because it is not metabolised. Conversely, when oestrogen levels are low, FAAH is not downregulated, and therefore anandamide is metabolised at the usual rate. This would account for the up and down moods in menopause as the levels of oestrogen go up and down. The ECS also plays a role in modulating oestrogen release by downregulating luteinising hormone (LH) in the pituitary and gonadotropin-releasing hormone (GnRH) from the hypothalamus. The ECS downregulates the hypothalamic-pituitary-ovarian (HPO) axis by reducing GnRH and LH, which leads to reduced oestrogen levels. The other half of the equation is that oestrogen downregulates FAAH and thus increases anandamide levels. Progesterone is also regulated to some extent by the ECS.

The ECS has control over LH release and therefore influences ovulation. Once ovulation occurs, the corpus luteum produces progesterone which seems also to downregulate FAAH, which increases anandamide (Gorzalka & Dang, 2012). Anandamide is higher during the follicular phase (the first half) of the menstrual cycle, and even higher during ovulation, but is lower during the luteal phase (the second half) of the menstrual cycle. Even in fertility and pregnancy the level of anandamide is low to allow for implantation and for continuing the pregnancy, but then a surge of anandamide facilitates labour.

There is a two-way process. Oestrogen modulates CB1 and CB2 receptors and the production and degradation of anandamide in both the CNS and the periphery. Conversely, the ECS downregulates the production of oestrogen by reducing the release of GnRH.

During menopause the levels of oestrogen and progesterone are low, therefore FAAH is not downregulated. Anandamide continues to be metabolised at a faster rate, leading to the various signs and symptoms of menopause such as insomnia, mood swings, emotional responses such as anxiety and depression, low libido, bone loss and weight gain. Using CBD makes sense in menopause, as the CBD downregulates the FAAH thus restoring balance to the levels of anandamide.

Hot flushes are a distressing symptom of menopause for many women. While anecdotally CBD seems to have some effect, this has not yet been supported by clinical studies. How *could* CBD help hot flushes?

One possible mechanism is that, as we have seen earlier, CBD can influence the serotonin receptor. Why is this relevant? Conventionally, one of the non-hormonal methods of dealing with hot flushes is an SSRI antidepressant (Shams et al., 2014) which blocks the reuptake of serotonin into neurons. In the same way, CBD may help hot flushes by stimulating serotonin receptors.

Part 3
Safety Considerations
and Summary

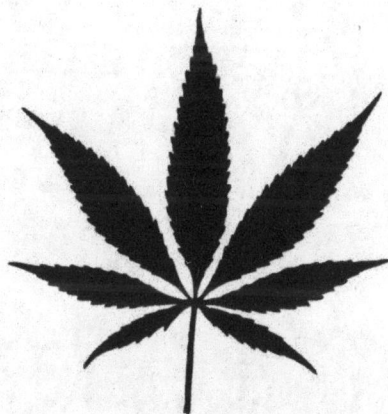

Chapter 21

The Safety of CBD

To the time of writing the consensus is that CBD oil is safe, with very few side effects.

Although the question about safety of CBD often arises, any practitioner can confidently say that its safety is confirmed by the now large body of literature providing clinical evidence of its safety and efficacy. The one proviso is that there is the potential for CBD-pharmaceutical interactions. This will be discussed later in the chapter.

The following graph (Gable, 2006) compares the safety of cannabis with other commonly used substances.

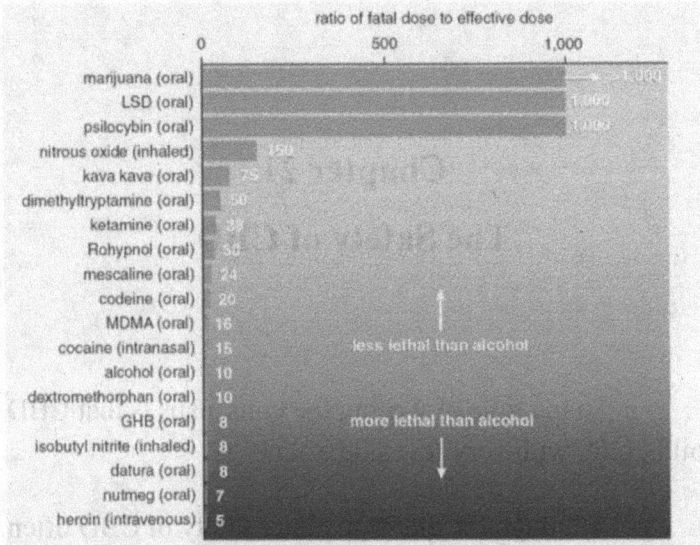

ratio of fatal dose to effective dose

	0	500	1,000
marijuana (oral)			>1,000
LSD (oral)			1,000
psilocybin (oral)			1,000
nitrous oxide (inhaled)	150		
kava kava (oral)	75		
dimethyltryptamine (oral)	50		
ketamine (oral)	38		
Rohypnol (oral)	30		
mescaline (oral)	24		
codeine (oral)	20		
MDMA (oral)	16		
cocaine (intranasal)	15	less lethal than alcohol	
alcohol (oral)	10		
dextromethorphan (oral)	10		
GHB (oral)	8	more lethal than alcohol	
isobutyl nitrite (inhaled)	8		
datura (oral)	8		
nutmeg (oral)	7		
heroin (intravenous)	5		

American Scientist, 2006

Lachenmeier and Rehn (2015) compared the risks of alcohol, tobacco, cannabis, and other illicit drugs using the margin of exposure (MOE) approach. The MOE is defined as the *"ratio between toxicological threshold (benchmark dose) and estimated human intake."* The study showed that alcohol, nicotine, cocaine, and heroin fall into the high-risk category with MOE <10. The rest of the compounds fall into a risk category with an MOE < 100. Cannabis falls into a category on its own of an MOE >10,000.

Cannabis has been used for centuries. However, there are always some concerns regarding long-term use. While the historical record seems to show long-term safety, there are few scientific studies. The few longitudinal studies that have been done evaluated the use of CBD in children with drug-resistant epilepsy, Dravet syndrome. CBD was given as an add-on in high doses of 25-50 mg/kg/day (Laux et al., 2020; Park et al., 2019).

In the short-term any minor side effects, such as those listed below, are generally mentioned.

- **Dry mouth** - commonly called *cottonmouth* can be annoying but is not dangerous. It can be relieved by drinking more water.

- **Drowsiness** - as one of the uses of CBD is for insomnia, to help people to sleep, drowsiness may be considered a side effect or a direct effect and one of the reasons it is used. This can be dose dependent. A solution to this, if you are experiencing excess drowsiness, is to take the dose at night.

- **Low blood pressure** - is not uncommon and can lead to the next symptom – light-headedness. In one study (Jadoon, Tan, & O'Sullivan, 2017), when a group of healthy volunteers was given an acute single dose of CBD, they showed a drop in blood pressure (BP), and a drop in blood pressure related to stress. However, in a longitudinal study

(Sultan, O'Sullivan, & England, 2020), the effect was lost as the participants developed tolerance, although the BP reduction related to stress persisted. The CBD seems to protect the body from high BP due to stress. The mechanism through which this occurs is thought to be due to reduction of arterial stiffness and improvements in endothelial function. Using CBD to treat hypertension many not necessarily be a primary treatment, but if you are taking CBD and BP does improve, then medication can be reduced and all in all it probably is a good thing.

– **Decreased appetite** -THC is well known to produce the *munchies* while CBD seems to reduce appetite. A study in rats (Farrimond, Whattey, &Williams, 2012), showed that CBD could decrease appetite. This weight loss also occurs in human cannabis users (Clark et al., 2018). So, is it a side effect? Or, since obesity is a big problem today, it is not certain whether weight loss should be considered a side effect or a positive effect?

– **Gut issues** - some may suffer gut side effects, but they are generally mild and temporary. This is probably related to dosage. It is noteworthy that generally CBD has been shown to have a positive effect on the gut.

–   **Liver issues** - while liver damage occurred in a study where mice were given high doses of CBD. The product used in this study was Epidiolex, a CBD isolate without terpenes. We have seen previously that CBD on its own (i.e., without terpenes) can be more dangerous. In humans, the maximum dose of Epidiolex is 20 mg/kg/day. In these studies doses of up to 2,460 mg/kg for acute dosing and 615 mg/kg for subacute dosing for 10 days were used. (Ewing et al., 2019) I should point out that very high doses of any substance can cause damage. Damage does not seem to occur in normal doses, and it is notable that CBD has been shown to treat liver damage.

–   **Lung issues** - these can be a problem, especially if the cannabis is being smoked. In this book I have only discussed CBD oil, but for completeness I will mention smoking cannabis. CBD oil is not generally used for smoking although some do vape their CBD oil. There is concern that smoking cannabis may cause lung cancer. There is no evidence that smoking cannabis causes lung cancer, and it is more likely that it does not (Huang et al., 2015). Should there be a risk, I consider it would still be lower than with tobacco smoke. The factors to consider are concomitant smoking of tobacco, and length and heaviness of use. Of course, with prolonged use, a heavy cannabis smoker, especially if also smoking tobacco at the same time, would run a greater risk of lung cancer than if smoking small amounts of cannabis only. Generally, MC is given via an oral route, not inhaled, so there is no chance of lung cancer. In fact, the CBD component of cannabis has been shown to have a therapeutic option for treatment of highly invasive lung cancers (Ramer et al., 2012).

When considering the validity of outcomes of studies, there are several things to consider. The group of people being studied will influence the outcome, for example, in the USA cannabis was classed as a narcotic, therefore research was difficult. Whether quality-controlled CBD oil was used. Some studies looked at heavy cannabis smokers using illicit cannabis. The dosage of the substance is also important, as are the origins of the cannabis used in the study; how it was grown; whether pesticides were used, and whether there were heavy metals in the soil will also make a difference. Quality control is important. Also, some of the studies were based on synthetic cannabis product use, and as we have already seen, SCs do have more side effects than the natural product.

In one study *"the most commonly reported side effects were tiredness, diarrhea, and changes of appetite and weight."* The researchers (Iffland & Grotenherrmen,

2017) also commented that CBD had a better side effect profile that pharmaceuticals that were used to treat these medical conditions. The outcome of yet another recent study (Larsen & Shahinas, 2020) was that *"overall the administration was well tolerated with mild side effects."*

Just as it is important to consider the validity of studies that have been carried out, it is important to consider what you read on the Internet. A recent article citing a study by Vozoris et al. (2021) looked at morbidity and mortality associated with prescription cannabinoid drug use in COPD. The researchers neglected to consider the fact that SCs were used in the study. As a result, the headline of the online article, Cannabinoids Associated with Negative Respiratory Health (2021), gives a false impression by suggesting that cannabinoid use is dangerous for people with COPD.

A spate of fifty-two deaths in the USA was mistakenly attributed to CBD oil. Investigation found CBD oil was not the cause of the deaths. The product these people were using was a synthetic cannabinoid – 4-Cyano CUMYL-BUTINACA (4-CCB), (mis)labelled as CBD oil (Horth et al., 2018).

MC is safe to give to cancer patients for palliative reasons. MC has been shown to help with sleep, pain, weakness, nausea, and lack of appetite. Schleider et al.

(2018) were confident that *"cannabis as a palliative treatment for cancer patients seems to be a well-tolerated, effective and safe option to help patients cope with the malignancy related symptoms."*

In a report of the Expert Committee on Drug Dependence (2018), the WHO stated that CBD is safe. So, overall, natural CBD is safe, and the side effects (if any) are generally rare and mild and do settle with time or with dose modification!

The one proviso

The one issue that we must consider is CBD-pharmaceutical drug interactions. We know that CBD has a competitive inhibiting effect on the cytochrome P450 enzymes, notably CYP 3A4 and CYP 2DC (Zendulka et al., 2016). Competitive inhibition means that the CBD occupies the site of enzymic activity and prevents other compounds being metabolised.

CYP 3A4 and CYP 2DC are also the main cytochrome P450 enzymes that metabolise pharmaceuticals, although there are others. When CBD is taken, these enzymes are competitively inhibited, and any concomitant pharmaceuticals being taken may have their metabolism compromised. In other words, these pharmaceuticals will remain in the body, unmetabolized and therefore, their activity will be sustained, and/or drug levels could increase and become toxic, which can lead to problems. For example, if the person is on a BP medication, it may not be metabolised, and medication blood levels rise. They may start to feel dizzy because BP drops and may drop too low. A simple solution is to reduce the dose of the BP medication. An important point to make here is that not everyone has the same enzymes, as the cytochrome enzymes have a great variability due to polymorphisms. Some people are just more sensitive than others based on their individual genetic makeup.

Which drugs could be affected?

The following list accounts for most of the pharmaceuticals currently in use and includes antihistamines, antiretrovirals, antipsychotics, beta blockers, benzodiazepines, calcium channel blockers, cyclosporine, haloperidol, macrolides, opioids, sildenafil, statins (atorvastatin and simvastatin but not pravastatin and rosuvastatin), SSRIs, tricyclic antidepressants.

However – there is always a *however* - the inhibition of cytochrome P450 enzymes only happens with high doses of CBD and not with normal doses.

Neurologists tend to use high doses in paediatric seizure patients (Dravet syndrome), where doses as high as 25-50 mg CBD/kg are used. Here, children on clobazam, an anti-epileptic, and CBD, showed clobazam toxicity due to cytochrome P450 interaction. Levels of clobazam need to be monitored and doses reduced if toxicity develops (Chang, 2019).

In other patients, the CBD dose is generally in the range of 0.25 - 5 mg/kg of CBD. Even in this low range, some adverse effects may be seen but is much less likely. The best course of action is to monitor the patient. This can be done clinically by measuring the BP and reducing the dose if the BP is getting too low. With some drugs, serum levels can be monitored by doing blood tests. I would strongly recommend that patients on both CBD and pharmaceuticals have regular medical check-ups.

Is CBD safe in pregnancy?

There are many symptoms in pregnancy that can make this time difficult, such as nausea, sleeping problems, back pain, and appetite problems. CBD has been shown to help these symptoms, *but* is CBD safe in pregnancy?

We saw earlier that anandamide plays a role in pregnancy. A low anandamide is needed for implantation and for continuing the pregnancy. A high anandamide seems to trigger labour. Giving CBD may raise anandamide levels and cause a miscarriage.

In Persia, around 600 BCE, the Zoroastrian text, *Zend Avesta*, considered cannabis as a prohibitive herb as it could cause abortions.

Researchers who studied illicit cannabis use in pregnant women discovered intrauterine growth retardation in the foetus (El Marroun et al., 2009). The article describing the study, mentioned the women were using illicit cannabis, therefore, it may be assumed they were using or smoking marijuana. The results of an earlier study (Hurd et al., 2005) showed that marijuana use in pregnant women impairs growth in mid-gestation foetuses.

The discussion following a study carried out later by Jaques et al. (2014), again highlights a negative impact on development. They stated, *"current evidence indicates that cannabis use, both during pregnancy and lactation, may adversely affect neurodevelopment, especially during periods of critical brain growth both in the developing fetal brain and during adolescent maturation, with impacts on neuropsychiatric, behavioural and executive functioning."* However, again the discussion is about cannabis, possibly illicit cannabis with THC, and presumably smoked, and not specifically about using CBD oil.

According to Feinshtein et al. (2013), CBD can alter P- glycoprotein (P-gp) and breast cancer resistant protein (BCRP) expression in the human placenta and, therefore, reduce placental protective functions, which obviously is not good for the foetus.

CBD inhibits angiogenesis. This may be useful in treating cancer but is this good in pregnancy? CBD has been shown to be anti-angiogenic to human umbilical vein endothelial cells (Solinas et al., 2012).

There are limited studies showing safety of CBD in pregnancy (Sarrafpour et al., 2020). Considering the above discussion, the best course of action is not to use CBD oil during pregnancy.

One possibility is to use CBD oil or cream topically. CBD topically only affects the ECS of the skin and does not enter the bloodstream. Other forms of therapy such as acupuncture, massage, or gentle manipulation would be ideal and safe.

What about PEA?

One of the main features of PEA is its safety. The concern is whether it is safe in pregnancy.

PEA has been found to be safe in that it did not produce any genotoxic effects in human cells. This same paper also discussed studies in pregnant mice which showed no teratogenic or embryogenic effects (Nestman, 2016).

PEA was first discovered over fifty years ago, and since then there have been no significant effects noted. As PEA is naturally made by the body, it probably is safe during pregnancy, however, formal studies and clinical evidence of its safety would give peace of mind.

When PEA was given to pregnant rats at very high doses of 250, 500, or 1,000 mg/kg bodyweight, the researchers found no abnormalities in the pups (Deshmukh, Gumaste, Subah, & Bogoda, 2021). General human dosage is in the order of 8-30 mg/kg/day. It is not known whether the results of this study are transferable to pregnant women as more research is needed. However, studies like this add to the safety data.

Doing studies on pregnant women is fraught with danger and probably would not be approved. The best practice always, is to avoid all drugs, herbs, and nutraceuticals, during pregnancy, unless absolutely necessary.

If in doubt – don't!

If, however, some treatment is needed during pregnancy, then PEA would be a possible choice, as well as using modalities such as topical CBD, acupuncture, massage, or gentle manipulation.

Caution - do not mix CBD with alcohol

When researchers, Consroe, Carlini, Zwicker and Lacerda (1979), studied the effects of alcohol, alcohol plus CBD, and CBD alone on motor and psychomotor performances, they concluded that *"compared to placebo, alcohol and alcohol plus CBD, but not CBD alone, produced significant impairment of motor and psychomotor performances, overestimations of time production and subjective responses indicating an inaccurate self-perception of their intoxication and deficits."* This study was done with a relatively large dose of CBD. The 200 mg dose reduced the blood alcohol level. No studies have been done to ascertain whether a smaller dose would be effective. Anecdotally, there is no significant effect with the large dose, although some do feel extra drowsy and there may be a slight drop in BP causing light-headedness.

CBD has been shown to protect the body from excessive use of alcohol. CBD reduces liver damage, protects against fatty liver disease, is an antioxidant, and a neuroprotectant. It also can reduce the hang-over, BUT that is not a reason to mix!

However, the mixing of alcohol and THC does increase levels of blood THC. This study (Hartman et al., 2015) was carried out using vaporised cannabis. The chance of fatal motor vehicle accidents is greatly increased when alcohol and THC are mixed (Chihuri, Li, & Chen, 2017).

Chapter 22

How to Use CBD

Before we discuss the various ways of using CBD, it is important to consider bioavailability. Bioavailability is the degree to which a drug becomes available to the body. How much CBD gets into the bloodstream depends on dose and route of taking. The method used affects speed of onset and duration of the effects of CBD.

The most common ways of taking CBD oil are:

1. orally,

2. topically, and

3. inhaled – vaped.

Other routes that are not so popular include rectal, in suppository form, which is a good way to administer for gut problems, and vaginal pessaries, usually used for gynaecological conditions. One suggestion is to soak a tampon in CBD oil, then insert.

The most common method is to take the oil orally. There are several forms this can take such as oil, capsule, or even a gummie (not yet available in Australia). Anything that goes into the mouth, (food, drugs, CBD oil) and is swallowed ends up in the stomach. Stomach acid and enzymes start to metabolise whatever has been swallowed, then what remains is absorbed and goes straight to the liver. Here, the first pass effect takes place; this means that the liver breaks down a large portion of the absorbed drug or CBD before it reaches the main blood stream.

The main CBD metabolite is 7-hydroxycannabidiol (7 OH-CBD) which is further metabolised to 7-carboxy-cannabidiol (7-COOH-CBD, which is excreted in the faeces and urine.

Oral edibles such as gummies have an exceptionally low bioavailability of approximately 4-20%. Experiments in dogs (Samara, Bialer, & Mechoulan,1988) showed the figure of 20% and this is largely due to the first pass effect.

Eating CBD then, is not necessarily a good option. However, when taken with food, CBD is absorbed three to five times better than on an empty stomach. Taking the CBD with fatty food such as avocado, fish, and nuts, will help even more (Millar, Stone, Yates' O'Sullivan. 2018). Indeed, CBD bioavailability increases fourfold with a high fat meal, which enhances the potential of the CBD to be also absorbed through the gut enteric lymphatic system (Perucca & Bialer, 2020).

Piperine, found in black pepper, increases absorption of CBD. Izgelov, Domb, and Hoffman (2020) found that adding piperine to CBD increased oral bioavailability two-and -a -half-fold. One component of black pepper is beta-caryophyllene, one of the terpenes, which may also enhance the entourage effect.

Another way around this is to take a bigger dose so that more gets into the bloodstream. Although this may not be an advisable option! The onset of action takes about two hours, but the effect may last longer. When compared with smoked or vaped cannabis, the effect is very quick but lasts a shorter time.

The sublingual route is an effective oral method of taking CBD. The CBD oil is held in the mouth and under the tongue for a few minutes before swallowing; this allows some of the CBD to enter the blood stream through the mucous membranes of the mouth and thus avoid the first pass effect. Sublingual CBD has a quicker onset of action, with some feeling effects within twenty minutes. This is possibly because it has a significantly higher bioavailability (from 12 - 35%), than other oral methods of taking CBD. A study in rabbits demonstrated the increased bioavailability of the sublingual route (Mannila, Järvinen, Järvinen, & Jarho, 2007).

Smoking and vaping have a fast onset of action as the large surface area of the lungs helps to absorb the CBD, but the downside is that the duration of action is much shorter. Using the vaping route may be useful in the acute situation because of the fast onset of action. The inhalation route has been demonstrated to have a bioavailability of 34-46%, and even up to 50% (Huestis, 2007).

Another possibility is to use a nebuliser. This is a machine designed to deliver medications to the body through the lungs and is an essential item for most asthmatics. Nebulisers can produce a peak blood level of a medication in approximately thirty-six minutes (Millar, Stone, Yates, & O'Sullivan, 2018).

As mentioned earlier, CBD oil can be put into your hot cup of tea and the steam inhaled as you drink your tea.

The third method of using CBD oil is the topical route. The method is to rub or massage the oil or cream into the skin, into the area of concern. A topical application can be used for skin diseases such as eczema and psoriasis, and for Dupuytren's contractures, as well as for localised pain due to arthritis, injuries, and even just for muscle soreness after sport or activity. One important point is that topical CBD oil does not enter the bloodstream; the CBD works locally on the endocannabinoid system of the skin, and in the surrounding area. When CBD was applied to the skin it reduced joint swelling in an arthritis model study on rats (Hammell et al., 2016).

A fourth method is via rectal suppositories or even vaginal pessaries. Historically vaginal pessaries were mentioned in the ancient Egyptian papyrus as being useful for women's diseases. Rectal suppositories can be made up by compounding pharmacists.

The rectum has three drainage veins, the superior, middle, and inferior rectal veins. The superior rectal vein drains into the inferior mesenteric vein and then to the portal vein, and into the liver which means that some of the rectally absorbed CBD can have a partial first pass effect.

The middle and inferior rectal veins bypass the liver and the first pass effect by draining directly into the inferior vena cava. The moral of this story is that if you are using CBD suppositories, then do not insert them too high.

Huestis (2007) showed that rectally administered THC had twice the bioavailability of oral dosage due mainly to a higher absorption and a lower first pass effect metabolism. Although this was for THC, it is very likely possible to extrapolate the results to CBD use. The results of a mouse study (Schicho, & Storr, 2012), where the mouse was treated for induced colonic inflammation, showed significantly reduced inflammation with the use of rectal CBD, and no effect with oral CBD.

Rectal CBD is possibly useful for any form of gut inflammation, although this route is not for everyone.

Protocol

Every person is different, and treatment must be individualised. Therefore, it is hard to determine what dose of CBD is appropriate. The common adage, *Start Low and Go Slow*, is, perhaps, a good motto for CBD use. We can add to this adage, *Stay Low!*

Start Low-Go Slow-Stay Low

When considering how to use CBD, nothing can be simpler than the above adage.

The strength of the compounded CBD oil is 100 mg per millilitre. Generally, a graduated syringe, 0.1ml amounts, is supplied.

So, start low, with 0.1 ml daily, then increase slowly; every 3-4 days increase by 0.1 ml until you start to feel benefit, then remain at that dose. Taking more than the dose you feel well at will not necessarily improve things.

CBD can be taken daily or twice daily. For sleep issues, the dose is best taken at night.

In the case of anxiety, an extra 0.1-0.2 ml can be taken when anxiety develops. Once the anxiety is much improved, the CBD can be stopped and then taken on an as needed basis.

Deprescribing

Deprescribing is the term used for reducing any pharmaceutical that is being taken concurrently with the CBD. Once there is improvement in symptoms, then the pharmaceuticals can be slowly reduced.

Do not suddenly stop all pharmaceuticals when starting CBD or PEA.

Another reason for deprescribing is because of the influence of CBD on the cytochrome P450 enzymes as discussed earlier. Some medications may need to be reduced because the pharmaceuticals are not being metabolised.

***

Does CBD Work for Everyone?

The simple answer is, no! Nothing is one hundred percent effective. Perhaps the question we should ask is, *"Are there any reasons why CBD may not work for some people?"* Clearly, the answer is, yes, there are reasons. However, even when investigating the why, it is not possible to find answers for everyone; there will always be some unknowns.

Following are some of the reasons CBD may not be effective.

1. The source of the product is very important. Is the CBD ordered online, from the USA? Or is it from someone down the road, or from an acquaintance of a friend of a friend? Please be careful about your source. These products are unregulated and probably are not tested for purity or dosage, so you simply do not know what you are getting. If you obtain your CBD from a regulated reputable source, such as a compounding pharmacy, then you can be assured that the product is pure and the dosage as per the label is correct.

2. Everyone is different. Everyone needs a different dose; body size and age can be important, as well as if you have sensitivities or allergies. This is the

227

rationale for *start low and go slow*. Keep increasing the dose until there is benefit. Of course, if after a *reasonable* dose there is no improvement, there may be other issues present. Although what is reasonable can be subjective, most people, with rare exceptions, do not need more than 150 to 200 mg CBD. If 200mg is exceeded with minimal benefit, the possibility of other issues should be explored. As we have already discussed in the section on bioavailability, how you take your dose is also important; whether you take it orally or sub-lingually, with fatty food, or whether you smoke, vape, or nebulise, all these can make a difference.

3. You may have developed tolerance. If you have been smoking cannabis for some time before starting CBD, or if you have been taking high doses of CBD then it is possible that you have developed tolerance. Some people are unaware they have been taking high doses of CBD, especially if they are using an unregulated product. To overcome this, it may be necessary to take a one, or two-week break, a *cannabis holiday*, then restart at a lower dose.

4. You may have a genetic SNP that affects how your body uses CBD. As seen earlier, there are many SNPs affecting the ECS, which means that

there are many people in the population that have a SNP. With some SNPs CBD may work normally, while with others, CBD may not be as effective and/or produce side effects. "... *a set of candidate genes can be chosen which variants may determine the therapeutic effect and also the occurrence of possible side effects and adverse reactions"* (Hryhorowicz et al., 2018).

5. Women may be more sensitive to CBD than men. The menstrual cycle can play a role. Oestrogen levels have a bearing on the effect of cannabis, especially THC, but the situation is not quite so clear with CBD.

6. CBD does not work overnight. The person's expectation is important. Give it time and do not have unrealistic expectations. Maximum effectiveness could take up to six weeks. CBD may be part of the solution, not necessarily the whole solution.

7. Diet is important. As discussed earlier, the omega 3 to omega 6 ratio is important. Too much omega 6 may affect the way CBD works. A change of diet to include fish oil or krill oil will make a difference, as will the use of hemp oil as it has a balanced omega 3: omega 6 ratio (Kim, Li, & Watkins, 2011).

CBD does not fix an unhealthy lifestyle.

***

If CBD and PEA are so good, can they be used together to be even better?

In the Cannabis Master Class, one of the lecturers said that if the CBD is not working adequately, then PEA can be added. There has been speculation that PEA could be considered a part of the entourage effect.

Tagne et al. (2021), using a mouse model, showed synergy between CBD (hemp oil extract), and PEA for acute and chronic pain. The diagram below is from that paper and explains it very well.

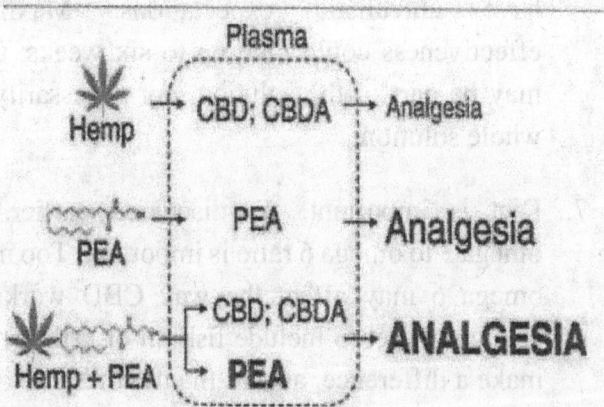

Synergy between CBD and PEA for
acute and chronic pain

One supplement company, released a product in September 2021, containing PEA, phytocannabinoids, and terpenes (available in the USA but not in Australia). The claim is that these three ingredients act synergistically and are part of the entourage effect. They achieve the same goals but via slightly different pathways (https://www.prnewswire.com/news-releases/metagenics-releases-hemp-advantage-plus-300940215.html accessed 16 Sep 2021).

Also, an Israeli biosciences company in Tel Aviv, announced a positive result in a trial of CBD and PEA late in 2021. The findings of these studies demonstrate that there is definitely synergy between CBD and PEA (https:// www. prnewswire.com/news-releases/therapix-biosciences-announces-positive-data-from-recent-pre-clinical-study-for-new-drug-candidate-thx-210-300938635.html accessed 16 Sep 2021).

My experience in clinical practice supports the evidence from the trials of the above companies.

However, it appears that the synergistic response between CBD and PEA is not always evident, that, in fact, in some cases, there may be antagonism between CBD and PEA. In a mouse model of MS, Rahini et al.

(2015) found that CBD worked well, and so did PEA, but when used together, the results were not as good as either alone. This means that more research is needed.

Chapter 23
Conclusion and Summary

The use of cannabis as a medicine dates back thousands of years. The ancient literature is filled with the positive benefits of cannabis. The prohibition laws of the1930s resulted in cannabis being considered an illicit drug, which negatively impacted on its use medicinally, while its illicit use increased. In the past twenty years, with researchers and doctors rediscovering the positive benefits of cannabis in many conditions and diseases, medicinal use is again becoming widespread. The resurgence of research, which has confirmed the safety and the benefits of cannabis as a medicine has played a big part in its acceptance.

This book outlines the use of cannabis, notably the use of CBD oil. As a sub-theme I have included a discussion of the use of palmitoylethanolamide (PEA), mainly for the benefit of those who cannot get CBD oil easily or cannot afford it.

The laws regarding CBD vary. Certainly, in Australia, approval to prescribe MC can be obtained through application to the TGA. However, an easier way is to prescribe compounded CBD, which is approved by the TGA as a Schedule 4 (S4) product, which means that any registered medical practitioner can prescribe it. Unfortunately, there are also state laws, and in Tasmania, until recently, the state law prohibited CBD prescriptions, even though it was legal in the other states. Prior to July 1st, 2021, the Tasmanian Government had its own cannabis scheme, the CAS, which commenced in 2017. This situation has now changed. From July 1st, 2021, doctors in Tasmania have been able to prescribe CBD oil without DoH approval.

The main issue now is the education of GPs in cannabis knowledge and prescribing.

As I live in Tasmania, I deliberately included the research on PEA, as CBD was not legally available when I first wrote this book. This situation has now changed.

Sources of CBD

One source is the illicit market. This was the primary source before the legalisation of MC. The danger here is that CBD purchased from unregulated sources is an unknown entity as far as the quality, contents, strength, and purity are concerned.

In states where the cannabis laws are more relaxed, and where there are cannabis clinics, these are a source of supply. The patient can ring a cannabis clinic in Queensland, have a phone consultation, and their prescription of CBD, or CBD/THC will be posted to them. This is legal. It was only illegal where a practitioner in Tasmania prescribed the same product prior to July 1st, 2021.

PEA has a very similar action as CBD. It is also cheaper and more freely available. There is now a supplement manufacturing company that is making a natural analgesic, where the only ingredient is PEA. This product is freely available over the counter.

The Federal Government and the TGA have now down-scheduled CBD from an S4 to an S3 product, which means it can be sold in pharmacies, over the counter, with no prescription required from a doctor. Initially the recommended maximum dose was 60 mg per day, but this was increased to 150 mg per day. This dosage is comparable to the doses used by my patients; my experience is that only a few of my patients needed doses greater than 150 mg per day. This regulation came into effect on February 1st, 2021, although that does not mean that CBD will be available soon. An S3 CBD product has not yet been approved, and this could take some time.

Ensuring safety when using CBD

The consensus is that if the TGA has approved CBD oil as an *over-the-counter* product, then it must be safe.

In principle, I do not support this. I agree that CBD is very safe. However, I don't believe that pharmacists will be able to give adequate advice and I would prefer that people see a doctor who is knowledgeable about CBD before starting use. This is another reason I have written this book – to educate the public and doctors about CBD.

Even though CBD is very safe, there still needs to be some supervision.

CBD and PEA can be used for many and varied conditions safely. Depending on the situation, it can be used as the sole treatment, although in many cases the patient is already on some form of pharmaceutical. Once CBD or PEA is started, the pharmaceutical can possibly be reduced in dose, or even totally de-prescribed, depending on response. It can be dangerous to abruptly stop the use of a pharmaceutical. The best pathway after starting CBD or PEA is to monitor, and slowly wean off the pharmaceuticals if, and as, the condition improves; this needs medical supervision. At the same time, other treatment modalities can be used, such as, acupuncture, nutrition, herbs, vitamins, and minerals.

More and more people are becoming suspicious of pharmaceuticals, and many are starting to opt for a more natural solution. The use of a natural herbal extract such as CBD oil is considered better and safer than a synthetic pharmaceutical. Many have chosen to consult naturopaths or acupuncturists for treatment rather than medical practitioners. However, now that there are doctors who practice integrative medicine, i.e., combine natural with conventional medicine, there is a move towards consulting these practitioners as they are likely to prescribe CBD or PEA.

CBD or PEA can be added to other treatments, although these are not necessarily a *magic bullet.*

While orthodox philosophy maintains that CBD should be a treatment of last resort, I totally disagree with this stance. It makes no sense to use a conventional treatment that could be more dangerous, e.g., opioids for chronic pain, when a safer product, CBD (or PEA), can be used first. Of course, where those many patients already on pharmaceuticals and suffering several side effects who wish to make a change, they should be able to do so, in a supported and supervised way. As mentioned above, the protocol would be that they start CBD or PEA and slowly wean off the pharmaceuticals.

The benefits of CBD are now well documented. That it is not for everyone, nor is it a panacea for all ills, is also well documented. It is not the *silver bullet* that many had hoped for. However, CBD has become the *flavour of the month*. An Internet search brings up a myriad of companies making and selling CBD products – not so much in Australia, but certainly in the USA. The hype is high, with each website, each company, saying their products are the best. Some of this hype is just that, hype! Hence, the importance of consulting with a practitioner who is knowledgeable about CBD and its uses.

Throughout this book I have attempted to highlight the importance of a wholistic approach to patient care. While CBD oil (and PEA) can be very helpful on their own, in other situations, they must be part of a broader approach to treatment and care. We should use all the tools in our toolbox to help people overcome their health issues. Do not rely only on CBD or PEA – always combine it with diet, lifestyle, exercise, nutrients, acupuncture, and other treatments and therapies that complement the PEA or CBD.

"If all you have is a hammer ... everything looks like a nail!"

Bernard Baruch (1870 -1965)

Hopefully the information in this book is useful. I have tried to include the latest research so that my narrative is supported by evidence-based scientific information.

CBD oil has been shown to be effective and safe – it truly is a Gift from Nature!

Part 4
References and
Resources

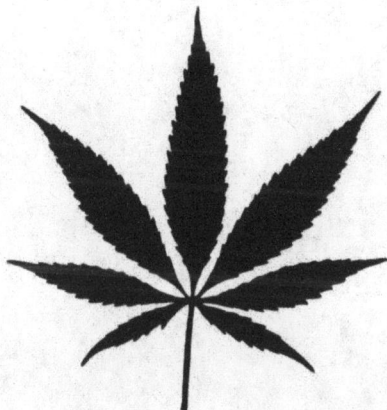

Part 1

An Introduction to Cannabidiol Oil

1. Introduction and background to use of medicinal cannabis

Habib,A., Okorokov, A., Hill, M., Bras, J., Lee, M., Li, ... Cox, J. (2019). Microdeletion in a FAAH pseudogene identified in a patient with high anandamide concentrations and pain insensitivity. *Br J Anaest, 123*(2), e249-e253. doi:10.1016/j.bja.2019.02.019

Compounding pharmacy. (n.d.) Retrieved from https://medical-dictionary.the freedictionary.com/compounding+pharmacy

Harris, J. (2021). GPs hold back on cannabis. Retrieved from https://tasmaniancountry.com/2021/10/16/gps-hold-back-on-cannabis/

Lynch, J. (2020). Cannabis is officially recognised as a medicine following historic vote. Retrieved from https://www.ladbible.com/news/latest-cannabis-is-now-officially-recognised-as-a-medicine-20201203

Courtney, S. (2021). Improvements to Tasmania's controlled access scheme for medicinal cannabis. Retrieved from https://premier.tas.gov.au/

2. What is CBD Oil?

Alger, B. (2013). Getting high on the endocannabinoid system. Cerebrum : the Dana forum on brain science, 2013,14.

Atakan, Z. (2012). Cannabis, a complex plant: Different compounds and different effects on individuals. *Ther Adv Psychopharmacol, 2*(6), 241-54. doi:10.1177/2045125312457586

Barrett, M., Scutt, A. & Evans,F. (1986). Cannflavin A and B, prenylated flavones from Cannabis sativa L. *Experientia, 42*(4), 452-3. doi:10.1007/BF02118655

Bolognini, D., Rock, E., Cluny, N., Cascio, M., Limebeer, C., Duncan, M., Stott, C., … Pertwee, R. (2013). Cannabidiolic acid prevents vomiting in Suncus murinus and nausea-induced behaviour in rats by enhancing 5-HT1A receptor activation. *Br J Pharmacol, 168*(6),1456-70. doi:10.1111/bph.12043

Brown, T. (2021). Equal driving laws for cannabis patients in Victoria. Retrieved from https://honahlee.com.au /articles /equal-driving-laws-cannabis-patients-victoria/

Cather, J., & Cather, J. C. (2020). Cannabidiol primer for healthcare professionals. *Proc (Bayl Univ Med Cent), 33*(3), 376-379. doi:10.1080/08998280.2020.1775437

Lafaye, G., Karila, L., Blecha, L., & Benyamina. A. (2017). Cannabis, cannabinoids, and health. *Dialogues Clin Neurosci, 19*(3), 309-316. doi:10.31887/DCNS.2017.19.3/glafaye

Lam, K., Ling, A., Koh, R., Wong, Y., & Say, Y. (2016). A review on medicinal properties of orientin. *Adv Pha rmacol Sci,* 2016, 4104595. doi: 10.1155/2016/4104595

Li, Y., Yao, J., Han, C., Yang, J., Chaudhry, M., Wang, S., ... Yin, Y. (2016). Quercetin, inflammation and immunity. *Nutrients, 158*(3), 167. doi:10.3390/nu8030167

Panche, A., Diwan, D., & Chandra, S. (2016). Flavonoids: an overview. *J Nutr Sci, 5,* e47. doi:10.1017/jns.2016.41

Pellesi, L., Licata, M.,Verri, P., Vandelli, D., Palazzoli, F., Marchesi, F., ... Guerzoni, S. (2018).

Pharmacokinetics and tolerability of oral cannabis preparations in patients with medication overuse headache (MOH)-a pilot study. *Eur J Clin Pharmacol.* *74*(11), 1427-1436. doi:10.1007/s00228-018-2516-3

Ren, J., Lu, Y., Qian, Y., Chen, B., Wu, T., & Ji, G. (2019). Recent progress regarding kaempferol for the treatment of various diseases *Exp Ther Med, 18*(4), 2759-2776. doi:10.3892/etm.2019.7886

Rock, E. & Parker, L. (2013). Effect of low doses of cannabidiolic acid and ondansetron on LiCl-induced conditioned gaping (a model of nausea-induced behaviour) in rats. *Br J Pharmacol, 169*(3), 685-92. doi:10.1111/bph.12162

Rock, E., Limebeer, C., & Parker,L. (2018). Effect of cannabidiolic acid and Δ^9-tetrahydrocannabinol on carrageenan-induced hyperalgesia and edema in a rodent model of inflammatory pain. *Psychopharmacology (Berl), 235*(11), 3259-3271. doi:10.1007/s00213-018-5034-1

Takeda, S., Misawa, K., Yamamoto, I., Watanabe, K. (2008). Cannabidiolic acid as a selective cyclooxygenase-2 inhibitory component in cannabis. *Drug Metab Dispos.* *36*(9),1917-21. doi:10.1124/dmd.108.020909

Takeda, S., Okazaki, H., Ikeda, E., Abe, S., Yoshioka, Y., Watanabe, K., Aramaki, H.(2014). Down-regulation of cyclooxygenase-2 (COX-2) by cannabidiolic acid in human breast cancer cells. *J Toxicol Sci, 39*(5), 711-6. doi:10.2131/jts.39.711

Towell, N. & Fowler, M. (2020). Drivers using medicinal cannabis could get green light. Retrieved from https//www.theage.com.au/national/victoria/drivers-using-medicinal-cannabis-to-get-green-light-20201014-p564z0.html

Vincent, M. (2021). Father who juiced cannabis for sick daughters avoids jail. Retrieved from https://www.abc.net.au/news/2018-07-20/father-who-juiced-cannabis-for-sick-daughters-avoids-jail/9856976.html

Yan, X., Qi, M., Li, P., Zhan, Y., & Shao, H. (2017). Apigenin in cancer therapy: Anti-cancer effects and mechanisms of action. *Cell Biosci, 7,* 50. doi:10.1186/s13578-017-0179-x

Zagzoog, A., Mohamed, K., Kim, H., Kim, E., Frank, C., Black, T., … Laprairie, R. (2020). In vitro and in vivo pharmacological activity of minor cannabinoids isolated from Cannabis sativa. *Sci Rep, 10*(1), 20405. doi:10.1038/s41598-020-77175-y

Resources

Cannabis and your body. Retrieved from https://weedmaps.com/learn/cannabis-and-your-body/difference-between-thca-thc.pdf

Weedmaps. Retrieved from https://weedmaps.com/learn/dictionary/cannabinoid/

CBD health and wellness (2020). Retrieved from https://cbdhealthandwellness.net/2020/04/25/what-are-flavonoids/

Saunders, N. Cannabidiolic acid (CBDA): The definitive guide. (2021, 29 October). Retrieved from https://wayofleaf.com/cannabis/ailments/cannabidiolic-acid-cbda

3. The Cannabis Plants

Sawler, J., Stout, J., Gardner, K., Hudson, D., Vidmar, J., Butler, L., … & Myles, S. (2015) The genetic structure of marijuana and hemp. *PLoS One*, *10*(8), e0133292. doi:10.1371/journal.pone.0133292

Resources

Hemp. (2020). In Britannica. Retrieved from https://www.britannica.com/plant/hemp.html

How to identify female and male marijuana plants. Retrieved from https://www.wikihow.com/Identify-Female-and-Male-Marijuana-Plants

Boshkova, M. (2021). Male cannabis plant: How to identify and use the male weed plant. Retrieved from https://www.highermentality.com/male-cannabis-plant/

Desjardins, J. (2018). The anatomy of a cannabis plant, and its lifecycle. Retrieved from https://www.visualcapitalist.com/anatomy-cannabis-plant/

4. Cannabis use throughout history

Reynolds, R. (1890) Therapeutical uses and toxic effects of cannabis indica. *Lancet, 135*(3473), 637-638. doi: https://doi.org/10.1016/S0140-6736(02)18723-X

Resources

Lyons, S. (2019, June 13). Cannabis traces from 2,500-year-old funeral braziers in China are earliest evidence of pot smoking. Retrieved from https://www.abc.net.au/news/science/2019-06-13/early-evidence-of-cannabis-smoking-found-in-china/11200414

Cannabis treatments in obstetrics and gynecology: A historical review. Retrieved from https://www.420magazine.com/community/threads/cannabis-treatments-in-obstetrics-and-gynecology-a-historical-review.155695/

Conrad, C. (1997). *Hemp for health.* Vermont, VA: Healing Arts Press.

Hua Tuo. New Word Encyclopedia. Retrieved from https://www.newworldencyclopedia.org/entry/Hua_Tuo

Mechoulam, R., & Hanu, L. (2001). The cannabinoids: An overview. Therapeutic implications in vomiting and nausea after cancer chemotherapy, in appetite promotion, in multiple sclerosis and in neuroprotection. *Pain Res Manage, 6*(2), 67-73.

Pain, S. (2015). A potted history. *Nature, 525*, S10–S11. https://doi.org/10.1038/525S10a

Perez, A. (2020). Queen Victoria used cannabis regularly for relief. Retrieved from https://thehighestcritic.com/blog/queen-victoria-used-cannabis-regularly-for-relief/

Russo, E. (2002). Cannabis treatments in obstetrics and gynecology: A historical review. *Journal of Cannabis Therapeutics,* 2(3-4), 5-35 https://doi.org/10.1300/J175v02n03_0

Sinclair, J. (2018). *Introduction to ethnopharmacology of cannabis: Medicinal cannabis education* [Course book]. Melbourne, Australia.

Branfalt, T. (2020 May 29). *Study identifies likely Cannabis use at ancient Israel site.* Retrieved from https://www.ganjapreneur.com/study-identifies-likely-cannabis-use-at-ancient-israel-site/

Wilcox, A. (2014, March 6). The origin of the word 'Marijuana'. Retrieved from https://www.leafly.com/news/cannabis-101/where-did-the-word-marijuana-come-from-anyway-01fb

5. The Endocannabinoid System

Devane, W., Hanus, L., Breuer, A., Pertwee, R., Stevenson, L., Griffin, G, ... Mechoulam, R. (1992). Isolation and structure of a brain constituent that binds to the cannabinoid receptor. *Science, 258*(5090),1946-9. doi:10.1126/science.1470919

Fride, E. (2004). The endocannabinoid-CB(1) receptor system in pre- and postnatal life. *Eur J Pharmacol, 500*(1-3), 289-97. doi:10.1016/j.ejphar.2004.07.033

Fride, E. (2008). Multiple roles for the endocannabinoid system during the earliest stages of life: pre- and postnatal development. *J Neuroendocrinol,* 20 Suppl 1, 75-81. doi:10.1111/j.1365-2826.2008.01670.x

Fride, E., Bregman, T., & Kirkham, T. (2005). Endocannabinoids and food intake: Newborn suckling and appetite regulation in adulthood. *Exp Biol Med (Maywood), 230*(4), 225-34. doi:10.1177/153537020523000401

Fuss, J., Bindila, L., Wiedemann, K., Auer, M., Briken,P., & Biedermann, S. (2017). Masturbation to orgasm stimulates the release of the endocannabinoid 2-arachidonoylglycerol in humans. *J Sex Med, 14*(11), 1372-1379. doi:10.1016/j.jsxm.2017.09.016

Gaoni, Y & R. Mechoulam, R (1964) Isolation, structure, and partial synthesis of an active constituent of hashish. *J Am Chem Soc, 86*(8), 1646–1647

Grant, I. & Cahn. B. (2005). Cannabis and endocannabinoid modulators: Therapeutic promises and challenges. *Clin Neurosci Res, 5*(2-4), 185-199. doi:10.1016/j.cnr.2005.08.015

Martínez-Peña, A., Lee, K., Petrik, J., Hardy, D., & Holloway, A. (2021). Gestational exposure to $\Delta\,^9$-THC impacts ovarian follicular dynamics and angiogenesis in adulthood in wistar rats. *J Dev Orig Health Dis,12*(6), 865-69. doi:10.1017/S2040174420001282

Siebers, M., Biedermann, S., Bindila, L., Lutz, B., & Fuss,J. (2021). Exercise-induced euphoria and anxiolysis do not depend on endogenous opioids in humans. *Psychoneuroendocrinology,126*, 105173. doi:10.1016/j.psyneuen.2021.105173

Wu, J., Gouveia-Figueira, S., Domellöf, M., Zivkovic, A., & Nording, M. (2016). Oxylipins, endocannabinoids, and related compounds in human milk: Levels and effects of storage conditions. *Prostaglandins Other Lipid Mediat, 122*, 28-36. doi:10.1016/j.prostaglandins.2015.11.002

6. What are the Functions of the ECS?

Cabral, G., Raborn, E., Griffin, L., Dennis, J., & Marciano-Cabral, F. (2008). CB2 receptors in the brain: Role in central immune function. *Br J Pharmacol, 153*(2), 240-51. doi:10.1038/sj.bjp.0707584

Russo, E. (2016) Clinical endocannabinoid deficiency reconsidered: Current research supports the theory in migraine, fibromyalgia, irritable bowel, and other treatment-resistant syndromes. *Cannabis Cannabinoid Res, 1*(1), 154-165. doi:10.1089/can.2016.0009

Resources

Alger, B. (2013). Getting high on the endocannabinoid system. *Cerebrum, 2013*, 14. eCollection.

Devinsky, O., Cilio, M., Cross, H., Fernandez-Ruiz, J., French, J., Charlotte Hill, C., ... Friedman, D. (2014). Cannabidiol: pharmacology and potential therapeutic role in epilepsy and other neuropsychiatric disorders. *Epilepsia, 55*(6), 791-802. doi:10.1111/epi.12631

Komorowski, J. & Stepień, H. (2007). The role of the endocannabinoid system in the regulation of endocrine function and in the control of energy balance in humans. [Article in Polish] *Postepy Hig Med Dosw (Online). 61*,99-105.

Lu, H., & Mackie, K. (2016). An introduction to the endogenous cannabinoid system. *Biol Psychiatry, 79*(7), 516-25. doi: 10.1016/j.biopsych.2015.07.028

7. Palmitoylethanolamide (PEA)

Briskey, D., Mallard, A., & Rao, A. (2020). Increased absorption of palmitoylethanolamide using a novel dispersion technology system (LipiSperse®). *J Nutraceuticals Food Sci, 5*(2:3). doi:10.36648/nutraceuticals.5.2.3

Di Marzo, V., Melck, D., Orlando, P., Bisogno, T., Zagoory, O., Bifulco,M., ... De Petrocellis, L. (2001). Palmitoylethanolamide inhibits the expression of fatty acid amide hydrolase and enhances the anti-proliferative effect of anandamide in human breast cancer cells. *Biochem J, 358*(Pt 1), 249-55. doi: 10.1042/0264-6021:3580249

Hesselink, J. (2013). Evolution in pharmacologic thinking around the natural analgesic palmitoylethanolamide: from nonspecific resistance to PPAR-α agonist and effective nutraceutical. *J Pain Res, 6*, 625-34. doi:10.2147/JPR.S48653

Hesselink, J., de Boer, T., & Witkamp, R. (2013). Palmitoylethanolamide: A natural body-own anti-inflammatory agent, effective and safe against influenza and common cold. *Int J Inflam,* 2013, 151028. doi:10.1155/2013/151028

Petrosino, S., & Di Marzo, V. (2017). The pharmacology of palmitoylethanolamide and first data on the therapeutic efficacy of some of its new formulations *Br J Pharmacol,* *174*(11), 1349-1365. doi:10.1111/bph.13580

Petrosino, S., Moriello, A., Cerrato, S., Fusco, M., Puigdemont, A., De Petrocellis, L., & Di Marzo, L. (2016). The anti-inflammatory mediator palmitoylethanolamide enhances the levels of 2-arachidonoyl-glycerol and potentiates its actions at TRPV1 cation channels. *Br J Pharmacol, 173*(7), 1154-62. doi:10.1111/bph.13084

Resources

Castelain, P. (2020, February 4).Palmitoylethanolamide (PEA) – Safe, legal and better alternative to CBD. Retrieved from https://medium.com/@pietercastelein/palmitoylethanol amide-pea-safe-legal-and-better-alternative-to-cbd-763652a0b29f

Gatti, A., Lazzari, M., Gianfelice, V., Di Paolo, A., Sabato, E., & Sabato, A. (2012). Palmitoylethanolamide in the treatment of chronic pain caused by different etiopathogenesis. *Pain Med, 13*(9), 1121-30. doi:10.1111/j.1526-4637.2012.01432.x

Maccarrone, M. (2017). Metabolism of the endocannabinoid anandamide: Open questions after 25 years. *Front Mol Neurosci, 10*,166. doi:10.3389/fnmol.2017.00166

8. Terpenes

Pamplona, F., da Silva, L., & Coan, A. (2018). Potential clinical benefits of CBD-rich *Cannabis* extracts over purified CBD in treatment-resistant epilepsy: Observational data meta-analysis. *Front Neurol, 9*, 759. doi:10.3389/fneur.2018.00759

Resources

Terpene. In Merriam-Webster. Retrieved from https://www.merriam-webster.com/dictionary/terpene

Terpenes : Learn how terpenes work synergistically with cannabinoids. (2022). Retrieved from

https://www.medicaljane.com/category/cannabis-classroom/terpenes/#introduction-to-terpenes

9. The Entourage Effect

Blasco-Benito, S., Seijo-Vila, M., Caro-Villalobos, M., Tundidor, I., Andradas, C., García-Taboada, E., ... Sánchez, C. (2018). Appraising the "entourage effect": Antitumor action of a pure cannabinoid versus a botanical drug preparation in preclinical models of breast cancer. *Biochem Pharmacol, 157*, 285-293. doi:10.1016/j.bcp.2018.06.025

Cogan, P. (2020). The 'entourage effect' or 'hodge-podge hashish': the questionable rebranding, marketing, and expectations of cannabis polypharmacy. *Expert Rev Clin Pharmacol,* *13*(8), 835-845. doi:10.1080/17512433.2020.1721281

Cohen, K., & Weinstein, A. (2018). Synthetic and non-synthetic cannabinoid drugs and their adverse effects:A review from public health prospective. *Front Public Health, 6,* 162. doi:10.3389/fpubh.2018.00162

Ferber, S., Namdar, D., Hen-Shoval, D., Eger, G., Koltai, Shoval, H., ... Weller, A. (2020). The "entourage effect": Terpenes coupled with cannabinoids for the treatment of mood disorders and anxiety disorders. *Curr Neuropharmacol,* *18*(2), 87-96. doi:10.2174/1570159X17666190903103923

Gallily, R., Yekhtin, Z., & Hanuš, L. (2015). Overcoming the bell-shaped dose-response of cannabidiol by using *Cannabis* extract enriched in cannabidiol. *Pharmacology & Pharmacy*, *6*(2), 75-85. doi:10.4236/pp.2015.62010

Koltai,H., & Namdar, D. (2020). Cannabis phytomolecule 'entourage': From domestication to medical use. *Trends Plant Sci*, *25*(10), 976-984. doi:10.1016/j.tplants.2020.04.007

Pamplona, F., da Silva, L., & Coan, A. (2018). Potential clinical benefits of CBD-rich*cannabis* extracts over purified CBD in treatment-resistant epilepsy: Observational data meta-analysis. *Front Neurol*, *9*, 759. doi:10.3389/fneur.2018.00759

Russo, E. (2019). The case for the entourage effect and conventional breeding of clinical cannabis: No "strain," no gain. *Front Plant Sci*, *9*, 1969. doi:10.3389/fpls.2018.01969

Santiago, M., Sachdev, S., J., McGregor, I., & Connor, M. (2019). Absence of entourage: Terpenoids commonly found in *Cannabis sativa* do not modulate the functional activity of Δ^9-THC at human CB_1 and CB_2 receptors. *Cannabis Cannabinoid Res*, *4*(3), 165-176. doi:10.1089/can.2019.0016

10. Cannabidiol Oil (CBD Oil)

Bachhuber, M., Saloner, B., Cunningham, C., & Barry, C. (2014). Medical cannabis laws and opioid analgesic overdose mortality in the United States, 1999-2010. *JAMA Intern Med, 174*(10), 1668-73. doi:10.1001/jamainternmed.2014.4005

Bakas, T., van Nieuwenhuijzen, P., Devenish, S., McGregor, S., Arnold, J., & M Chebib, M. (2017). The direct actions of cannabidiol and 2-arachidonoyl glycerol at GABA A receptors. *Pharmacol Res, 119*, 358-370. doi:10.1016/j.phrs.2017.02.022

Costa, B., Giagnoni, G., Franke, C., Trovato, A., & Colleoni, M. (2004). Vanilloid TRPV1 receptor mediates the antihyperalgesic effect of the nonpsychoactive cannabinoid, cannabidiol, in a rat model of acute inflammation. *Br J Pharmacol, 143*(2), 247-50. doi:10.1038/sj.bjp.0705920

Deutsch, D. (2016). A personal retrospective: Elevating anandamide (AEA) by targeting fatty acid amide hydrolase (FAAH) and the fatty acid binding proteins (FABPs). *Front Pharmacol, 7*, 370. doi:10.3389/fphar.2016.00370

Elmes, M., Kaczocha, M., Berger, W., Leung, K., Ralph, B.,Wang, L., ... Deutsch, D. (2015). Fatty acid-binding proteins (FABPs) are intracellular carriers for Δ9-tetrahydrocannabinol (THC) and cannabidiol (CBD). *J Biol Chem, 290*(14), 8711-21. doi:10.1074/jbc.M114.618447

Hurd, Y., Spriggs, S., Alishayev, J., Winkel, G., Gurgov, K., Kudrich, C., ... Salsitz, E. (2019). Cannabidiol for the reduction of cue-induced craving and anxiety in drug-abstinent individuals with heroin use disorder: A double-blind randomized placebo-controlled trial. *Am J Psychiatry, 176*(11),911-922. doi:10.1176/appi.ajp.2019.18101191

Kathmann, M., Flau, K., Redmer, A., Tränkle, C., & Schlicker, E. (2006). Cannabidiol is an allosteric modulator at mu-and delta-opioid receptors. *Naunyn Schmiedebergs Arch Pharmacol, 372*(5), 354-61. doi: 10.1007/s00210-006-0033-x

Whalley, B., Bazelot, M., Rosenberg, E., & Tsien, R. (2018). A role of GPR55 in the antiepileptic properties of cannabidiol (CBD). *Neurology, 90*(15 Supplement), 2.277.

Resources

How CBD works: CBD and cannabinoid receptors. (2019, September 25).Retrieved from https://thecbdinsider.com/knowledge-center/how-cbd-works-cbd-cannabinoid-receptors/

11. How to Improve the ECS Naturally

Ahmadalipour, A., Fanid, L., Zeinalzadeh, N., Alizadeh, M., Vaezi, H., Aydinlou, Z., & Noorazar, S. (2020). The first evidence of an association between a polymorphism in the endocannabinoid-degrading enzyme FAAH (FAAH rs2295633) with attention deficit hyperactivity disorder. *Genomics, 112*(2), 1330-1334. doi:10.1016/j.ygeno.2019.07.024

Argueta, D., & DiPatrizio, N. (2017). Peripheral endocannabinoid signaling controls hyperphagia in western diet-induced obesity. *Physiol Behav, 171*, 32-39. doi:10.1016/j.physbeh.2016.12.044

Benyamina, A., Kebir, O., Blecha, L., Reynaud, M., & Krebs, M. (2011) CNR1 gene polymorphisms in addictive disorders: A systematic review and a meta-analysis. *Addict Biol, 16*(1), 1-6. doi:10.1111/j.1369-1600.2009.00198.x

Brellenthin, G., Crombie, K., Hillard, C., & Koltyn, K. (2017). Endocannabinoid and mood responses to exercise in adults with varying activity levels. *Translational Journal of the ACSM, 2*(21), 138-145. doi:10.1249/TJX.0000000000000046

Brellenthin, A., Crombie, K., Hillard, C., & Koltyn, K. (2017). Endocannabinoid and mood responses to exercise in adults with varying activity levels. *Med Sci*

Sports Exerc, 49(8), 1688-1696. doi:10.1249/MSS.0000000000001276

Chmelikova, M., Pacal, L., Spinarova, L., & Vasku, A. (2015). Association of polymorphisms in the endocannabinoid system genes with myocardial infarction and plasma cholesterol levels. *Biomed Pap Med Fac Univ Palacky Olomouc Czech Repub, 159*(4), 535-9. doi:10.5507/bp.2014.043

Console-Bram, L., Marcu, J., & Abood, M. (2012). Cannabinoid receptors: nomenclature and pharmacological principles. *Prog Neuropsychopharmacol Biol Psychiatry, 38*(1), 4-15. doi:10.1016/j.pnpbp.2012.02.009

Doris, J., Millar, S., Idris, I., & O'Sullivan, S. (2019). Genetic polymorphisms of the endocannabinoid system in obesity and diabetes. *Diabetes Obes Metab, 21*(2), 382-387. doi:10.1111/dom.13504

Ehlers, C., Slutske, W., Lind, P., & Wilhelmsen, K. (2007). Association between single nucleotide polymorphisms in the cannabinoid receptor gene (CNR1) and impulsivity in southwest California Indians. *Twin Res Hum Genet, 10*(6), 805-11. doi:10.1375/twin.10.6.805

Escosteguy-Neto, J., Fallopa, P., Varela, P., Filev, R., Tabosa, A., & Santos-Junior, J. (2012).

Electroacupuncture inhibits CB1 upregulation induced by ethanol withdrawal in mice. *Neurochem Int, 61*(2), 277-85. doi:10.1016/j.neuint.2012.05.014

Felton, S., Kendall, A., Almaedani, A., Urquhart, P., Webb, A., Kift, R., ... Rhodes, L. (2017). Serum endocannabinoids and N-acyl ethanolamines and the influence of simulated solar UVR exposure in humans in vivo. *Photochem Photobiol Sci, 16*(4), 564-574. doi:10.1039/c6pp00337k

Frost, M., Nielsen, T., Wraae, K., Hagen, C.,Piters, E., & Beckers, S., ... Andersen, M. (2010). Polymorphisms in the endocannabinoid receptor 1 in relation to fat mass distribution. *Eur J Endocrinol, 163*(3), 407-12. doi:10.1530/EJE-10-0192

Guy, G., & Di Marzo, V. (2014). Care and feeding of the endocannabinoid system: A systematic review of potential clinical interventions that upregulate the endocannabinoid system. *PLoS One, 9*(3), e89566. doi:10.1371/journal.pone.0089566

Hanus, L., Avraham, Y., Ben-Shushan, D., Zolotarev, O., Berry, E., & Mechoulam, R. (2003). Short-term fasting and prolonged semistarvation have opposite effects on 2-AG levels in mouse brain. *Brain Res, 983*(1-2), 144-51. doi:10.1016/s0006-8993(03)03046-4

Hillard, C. (2014). Stress regulates endocannabinoid-CB1 receptor signaling. *Semin Immunol, 26*(5), 380-8. doi:10.1016/j.smim.2014.04.001

Hirvonen, J., Zanotti-Fregonara, P., Umhau, J., George, D.,Rallis-Frutos, D., Lyoo, C., ... Helig, M. (2013). Reduced cannabinoid CB1 receptor binding in alcohol dependence measured with positron emission tomography. *Mol Psychiatry, 18*(8), 916-21. doi:10.1038/mp.2012.100

Hirvonen, J., Zanotti-Fregonara, P., Gorelick, D., Lyoo, C., Rallis-Frutos, D., Morse, C., ... Innis, R. (2018). Decreased cannabinoid CB$_1$ receptors in male tobacco smokers examined with positron emission tomography. *Biol Psychiatry, 84*(10), 715-721. doi:10.1016/j.biopsych.2018.07.009

Hu, B., Bai, F., Xiong, L., & Wang, Q. (2017). The endocannabinoid system, a novel and key participant in acupuncture's multiple beneficial effects. *Neurosci Biobehav Rev, 77*, 340-357. doi:10.1016/j.neubiorev.2017.04.006

Klein, C., Hill, M., Chang, S., Hillard, C., & Gorzalka, B. (2012) .Circulating endocannabinoid concentrations and sexual arousal in women. *J Sex Med, 9*(6), 1588-601. doi:10.1111/j.1743-6109.2012.02708.x

Kong, X., Miao, Q., Lu, X., Zhang, Z., Chen, M., Zhang, J., Zhai, J. (2019). The association of endocannabinoid receptor genes (CNR1 and CNR2) polymorphisms with depression: A meta-analysis. *Medicine (Baltimore)*, *98*(46), e17403. doi:10.1097/MD.0000000000017403

Ligresti, A., Villano, R., Allarà, M., Ujváry, I., & Di Marzo, V. (2012). Kavalactones and the endocannabinoid system: The plant-derived yangonin is a novel CB_1 receptor ligand. *Pharmacol Res, 66*(2), 163-9. doi:10.1016/j.phrs.2012.04.003

MacDonald, I., & Chen, Y. (2021). The endocannabinoid system contributes to electroacupuncture analgesia. *Front Neurosci, 14*, 594219. doi:10.3389/fnins.2020.594219

Marcos, M., Pastor, I., de la Calle, C., Barrio-Real, L., Laso, F., & González-Sarmiento, R. (2012). Cannabinoid receptor 1 gene is associated with alcohol dependence. *Alcohol Clin Exp Res, 36*(2), 267-71. doi:10.1111/j.1530-0277.2011.01623.x

Milewicz, A., Tworowska-Bardzińska, U., Jędrzejuk, D., Lwow, F., Dunajska, K., Łaczmański, Ł., & Pawlak, M. (2011). Are endocannabinoid type 1 receptor gene (CNR1) polymorphisms associated with obesity and metabolic syndrome in postmenopausal Polish women?

Int J Obes (Lond), 35(3), 373-7. doi:10.1038/ijo.2010.145

Monteleone, P., Bifulco, M., Maina, G., Tortorella, A., Gazzerro, P., Proto, M., ... Maj, M. (2010). Investigation of CNR1 and FAAH endocannabinoid gene polymorphisms in bipolar disorder and major depression. *Pharmacol Res,* 61(5), 400-4. doi:10.1016/j.phrs.2010.01.002

Morena, M., Patel, S., Bains, J., & Hill, M. (2016). Neurobiological interactions between stress and the endocannabinoid system. *Neuropsychopharmacology,* 41(1), 80-102. doi:10.1038/npp.2015.166

Onaivi, E. (2010) Endocannabinoid system, pharmacogenomics and response to therapy. *Pharmacogenomics,* 11(7), 907-10. doi:10.2217/pgs.10.91

Pagano, C., Rossato, M., & Vettor, R. (2008). Endocannabinoids, adipose tissue and lipid metabolism. *J Neuroendocrinol,* 20 Suppl 1, 124-9. doi:10.1111/j.1365-2826.2008.01690.x

Peiró, A., García-Gutiérrez, M., Planelles, B., Femenía, T., Mingote, C., Jiménez-Treviño, L., ... Manzanares, J. (2020). Association of cannabinoid receptor genes (*CNR1 and CNR2*) polymorphisms and panic disorder. *Anxiety Stress Coping, 33*(3), 256-265. doi:10.1080/10615806.2020.1732358

Russo, E. (2016). Clinical endocannabinoid deficiency reconsidered: Current research supports the theory in migraine, fibromyalgia, irritable bowel, and other treatment-resistant syndromes. *Cannabis Cannabinoid Res, 1*(1), 154-165. doi:10.1089/can.2016.0009

Szejko, N., Fichna, J., Safranow, K., Żekanowski, C & Janik, P. (2020). Association of a variant of *CNR1* gene encoding cannabinoid receptor 1 with Gilles de la Tourette syndrome. *Front Genet, 11*,125. doi:10.3389/fgene.2020.00125

Part 2
Clinical Use of CBD Oil

12. Introduction

Bonn-Miller, M., Loflin, M., Thomas, B., Marcu, J., Hyke, T., & Vandrey R. (2017). Labeling accuracy of cannabidiol extracts sold online. *JAMA, 318*(17), 1708-1709. doi:10.1001/jama.2017.11909

Powell, D., Pacula, R., & Jacobson, M. (2018). Do medical marijuana laws reduce addictions and deaths related to pain killers? *J Health Econ, 58,* 29-42. doi:10.1016/j.jhealeco.2017.12.007

Reiman, A., Welty, M., & Solomon, P. (2017). Cannabis as a substitute for opioid-based pain medication: Patient self-report. *Cannabis Cannabinoid Res, 2*(1), 160-166. doi: 10.1089/can.2017.0012

Rønne, S., Rosenbæk, F., Pedersen, L., Frans Boch Waldorff, F., Nielsen, J., Riisgaard, H., & Søndergaard, J. (2021). Physicians' experiences, attitudes, and beliefs towards medical cannabis: A systematic literature review. *BMC Fam Pract, 22*(1), 212. doi:10.1186/s12875-021-01559-w

Scholl, L., Seth, P., Kariisa, M., Wilson, N., & Baldwin, G. (2018). Drug and opioid-involved overdose deaths— United States, 2013-2017. *MMWR Morb Mortal Wkly Rep, 67*(5152), 1419-1427. doi:10.15585/mmwr.mm675152e1

Zolotov, Y., Vulfsons, S., Zarhin, D., & Sznitman, S. (2018). Medical cannabis: An oxymoron? Physicians' perceptions of medical cannabis. *Int J Drug Policy, 57,* 4-10. doi:10.1016/j.drugpo.2018.03.025

13. Inflammatory Conditions

Abuhasira, R., Haviv, Y., Leiba, M., Leiba, A., Ryvo, L., & Novack, V. (2021). Cannabis is associated with blood pressure reduction in older adults: A 24-hours ambulatory blood pressure monitoring study. *Eur J Intern Med, 86,* 79-85. doi:10.1016/j.ejim.2021.01.005

Adejumo, A., Alliu, S., Ajayi, T., Adejumo, K., Adegbala, O., Onyeakusi, N., … Bukong, N. (2017). Cannabis use is associated with reduced prevalence of non-alcoholic fatty liver disease: A cross-sectional study. *PLoS One,* *12*(4), e0176416. doi:10.1371/journal.pone.0176416

Alhouayek, M. & Muccioli, G. (2014). Harnessing the anti-inflammatory potential of palmitoylethanolamide. *Drug Discov Today, 19*(10), 1632-9. doi:10.1016 /j.drudis.2014.06.007

Ali, A., & Akhtar, N. (2015). The safety and efficacy of 3% cannabis seeds extract cream for reduction of human cheek skin sebum and erythema content. *Pak J Pharm Sci, 28*(4), 1389-95.

Alswat, K. (2013). The role of endocannabinoids system in fatty liver disease and therapeutic potentials. *Saudi J Gastroenterol, 19*(4), 144-51. doi:10.4103/1319-3767. 114505

Anil, S., Shalev, N., Vinayaka, A., , S., Namdar, D., Belausov, E., ... Koltai, H. (2021). Cannabis compounds exhibit anti-inflammatory activity in vitro in COVID-19-related inflammation in lung epithelial cells and pro-inflammatory activity in macrophages. *Sci Rep, 11*(1), 1462. doi:10.1038/s41598-021-81049-2

Argueta, D., Ventura, C., Kiven, S., Sagi, V., & Gupta, K. (2020). A balanced approach for cannabidiol use in chronic pain. *Front Pharmacol, 11,* 561. doi:10.3389/fphar.2020.00561

Bachur, N., Masek, K., Melmon, K., & Udenfriend,S. (1965). Fatty acid amides of ethanolamide in mammalian tissue. *J Biol Chem, 240*, 1019-24.

Bhala, N., Emberson, J., Merhi, A., Abramson, S., Arber, N., Baron, J., ... Baigent, C. (2013). Vascular and upper gastrointestinal effects of non-steroidal anti-inflammatory drugs: meta-analyses of individual participant data from randomised trials. *Lancet, 382*(9894), 769-79. doi:10.1016/S0140-6736(13)60900-9

Blaskovich, M., Kavanagh, A., Elliott, A., Zhang, B., Ramu, S., Amado, M., ... Thurn, M. (2021). The antimicrobial potential of cannabidiol. *Commun Biol, 4*(1), 7. doi:10.1038/s42003-020-01530-y

Burstein, S. (2015). Cannabidiol (CBD) and its analogs: A review of their effects on inflammation. *Bioorg Med Chem, 23*(7), 1377-85. doi:10.1016/j.bmc.2015.01.059

Capano, A., Weaver, R., & Burkman, E. (2020). Evaluation of the effects of CBD hemp extract on opioid use and quality of life indicators in chronic pain patients: A prospective cohort study. *Postgrad Med, 132*(1), 56-61. doi:10.1080/00325481.2019.1685298

Costa, B., Giagnoni, G., Franke, C., Trovato, A., & Colleoni, M. (2004). Vanilloid TRPV1 receptor mediates the antihyperalgesic effect of the nonpsychoactive cannabinoid, cannabidiol, in a rat model of acute inflammation. *Br J Pharmacol, 143*(2), 247-50. doi:10.1038/sj.bjp.0705920

Couch, D., Cook, H., Ortori, C., Barrett, D., Lund, J., & O'Sullivan, S. (2019). Palmitoylethanolamide and cannabidiol prevent inflammation-induced hyperpermeability of the human gut in vitro and in vivo: A randomized, placebo-controlled, double-blind controlled trial. *Inflamm Bowel Dis, 25*(6), 1006-1018. doi:10.1093/ibd/izz017

Couch, D., Tasker, C., Theophilidou, E., Lund, J., & O'Sullivan, S. (2017). Cannabidiol and palmitoylethanolamide are anti-inflammatory in the acutely inflamed human colon. *Clin Sci (Lond), 131*(21), 2611-2626. doi:10.1042/CS20171288

Derakhshan, N., & Kazemi, M. (2016). Cannabis for refractory psoriasis—high hopes for a novel treatment and a literature review. *Curr Clin Pharmacol, 11*(2), 146-7. doi:10.2174/1574884711666160511150126

Esposito, E., & Cuzzocrea,S. (2013). Palmitoylethanolamide is a new possible pharmacological treatment for the inflammation associated with trauma. *Mini Rev Med Chem, 13*(2), 237-55.

Esposito, G., Pesce, M., Seguella, L., Sanseverino, W., Lu, J., Corpetti, C., & Sarnelli, G. (2020). The potential of cannabidiol in the COVID-19 pandemic. *Br J Pharmacol, 177*(21), 4967-4970. doi:10.1111/bph .15157

Gabrielsson, L., Mattsson, S., & Fowler, C. (2016). Palmitoylethanolamide for the treatment of pain: pharmacokinetics, safety and efficacy. *Br J Clin Pharmacol, 82*(4), 932-42. doi:10.1111/bcp.13020

Gatti, A., Lazzari, M., Gianfelice, V., Di Paolo, A., Sabato, E., & Sabato, A. (2012). Palmitoylethanolamide in the treatment of chronic pain caused by different etiopathogenesis. *Pain Med, 13*(9), 1121-30. doi:10.1111/j.1526-4637.2012.01432.x

Hammell, D., Zhang, L., Ma, F., Abshire, S., McIlwrath, S., Stinchcomb, A., & Westlund, K. (2016). Transdermal cannabidiol reduces inflammation and pain-related behaviours in a rat model of arthritis. *Eur J Pain, 20*(6), 936-48. doi:10.1002/ejp.818

Hawkey, C. (2001). COX-1 and COX-2 inhibitors. *Best Pract Res Clin Gastroenterol, 15*(5), 801-20. doi:10 .1053/bega.2001.0236

Hesselink, J., de Boer, T., & Witkamp, R. (2013). Palmitoylethanolamide: A body-own anti-inflammatory agent, effective and safe against influenza and common cold. *Int J Inflam, 2013,* 151028. doi:10.1155 /2013/151028.

Huang, L., Wang, L., Tan, J., Liu, H., & Ni, Y.,(2021). High-dose vitamin C intravenous infusion in the treatment of patients with COVID-19. *Medicine (Baltimore), 100*(19), e25876.doi:10.1097/MD.000000 0000025876

Iffland, K., & Grotenhermen, F. (2017). An update on safety and side effects of cannabidiol: A review of clinical data and relevant animal studies. *Cannabis Cannabinoid Res, 2*(1), 139-154. doi:10.1089/ can.2016 .0034

Kahlich, R., Klíma, J., Cihla, F., Franková, V., Masek, K., Rosický, M., ... Bruthans, J. (1979). Studies on prophylactic efficacy of N-2-hydroxyethyl palmitamide (Impulsin) in acute respiratory infections. Serologically controlled field trials. *J Hyg Epidemiol Microbiol Immunol, 23*(1), 11-24.

Karsak, M., Gaffal, E., Date, R., Wang-Eckhardt, L., Rehnelt, J., Petrosino, S., ... Zimner,A. (2007). Attenuation of allergic contact dermatitis through the endocannabinoid system. *Science, 316*(5830), 1494-7. doi:10.1126/science.1142265

Khodadadi, H., Salles, E., Jarrahi, A., Chibane, F., Costigliola, V.,Yu, J., ... Baban, B. (2020). Cannabidiol modulates cytokine storm in acute respiratory distress syndrome induced by simulated viral infection using synthetic RNA. *Cannabis Cannabinoid Res, 5*(3), 197-201. doi:10.1089/can.2020.0043

Lowe, H., Toyang, N., & McLaughlin, W. (2017). Potential of cannabidiol for the treatment of viral hepatitis. *Pharmacognosy Res, 9*(1), 116-118. doi:10.4103/0974-8490.199780

Lowin, T., Schneider, M., & Pongratz, G. (2019). Joints for joints: Cannabinoids in the treatment of rheumatoid arthritis. *Curr Opin Rheumatol, 31*(3), 271-278. doi:10.1097/BOR.0000000000000590

Marcum, Z., & Hanlon, J. (2010). Recognizing the risks of chronic nonsteroidal anti-inflammatory drug use in older adults. *Ann Longterm Care, 18*(9), 24-27.

Marini, I., Bartolucci, M., Bortolotti, F., Gatto, M., & Bonetti, G. (2012). Palmitoylethanolamide versus a nonsteroidal anti-inflammatory drug in the treatment of temporomandibular joint inflammatory pain. *J Orofac Pain, 26*(2), 99-104.

Monte, G., Soave, I., & Marci, R. (2013). Administration of micronized palmitoylethanolamide (PEA)-transpolydatin in the treatment of chronic pelvic pain in women affected by endometriosis: preliminary results. [Article in Italian]. *Minerva Ginecol, 65*(4), 453-63.

Nagarkatti, P., Pandey, R., Rieder, S., Hegde, V., & Nagarkatti, M. (2009). Cannabinoids as novel anti-inflammatory drugs. *Future Med Chem, 1*(7), 1333-49. doi:10.4155/fmc.09.93

Nguyen, L., Yang, D., Nicolaescu, V., Best, T., Ohtsuki, T., Chen, S., … Rosner, M. (2021). Cannabidiol inhibits SARS-CoV-2 replication and promotes the host innate immune response. *bioRxiv, 2021.03*.10.432967. doi: 10.1101/2021.03.10.432967 Preprint

Noce, A., Albanese, M., Marrone, G., Di Lauro, M., Zaitseva, A., Palazzetti, D., … Di Daniele, N. (2021). Ultramicronized palmitoylethanolamide (um-PEA): A new possible adjuvant treatment in COVID-19 patients. *Pharmaceuticals (Basel), 14*(4), 336.doi:10.3390/ph14040336

Norooznezhad, A., & Norooznezhad, F. (2017). Cannabinoids: Possible agents for treatment of psoriasis via suppression of angiogenesis and inflammation. *Med Hypotheses, 99*, 15-18. doi:10.1016/j.mehy.2016.12.003

Palmieri, B., Laurino, C., & Vadalà, M. (2019). A therapeutic effect of cbd-enriched ointment in inflammatory skin diseases and cutaneous scars. *Clin Ter, 170*(2), e93-e99. doi:10.7417/CT.2019.2116

Pandey, S., Kashif, S., Youssef, M., Sarwal, S., Zraik, H., Singh, R., & Rutkofsky, I. (2020). Endocannabinoid system in irritable bowel syndrome and cannabis as a therapy. *Complement Ther Med, 48*,102242. doi:10.1016/j.ctim.2019.102242

Pesce, M., Seguella, L., Cassarano, S., Aurino, L.Sanseverino, W., Lu,J., ... Esposito, G. (2020). Phytotherapics in COVID19: Why palmitoylethanolamide? *Phytother Res,* Dec 9. Online ahead of print. doi:10.1002/ptr.6978

Plesník, V., Havrlantová, M., J.,Januska, J., & Macková, O. (1977). Impulsin in the prevention of acute respiratory diseases in school children. [Article in Czech]. *Cesk Pediatr, 32*(6), 365-9.

Rajesh, M., Mukhopadhyay, P., Bátkai, S., Haskó, G., Liaudet, L., Drel, V., ... Pacher, P. (2007). Cannabidiol attenuates high glucose-induced endothelial cell inflammatory response and barrier disruption. *Am J Physiol Heart Circ Physiol, 293*(1), H610-9. doi:10.1152/ajpheart.00236.2007

Raso, G., Pirozzi, C., d'Emmanuele di Villa Bianca, R., Simeoli, R., Santoro, A., Lama, A., ... Meli, R. (2015). Palmitoylethanolamide treatment reduces blood pressure in spontaneously hypertensive rats: Involvement of cytochrome p450-derived eicosanoids and renin angiotensin system. *PLoS One, 10*(5), e0123602. doi:10.1371/journal.pone.0123602

Raso, G., Simeoli, R., Russo, R., Santoro, A., Pirozzi, C., d'Emmanuele di Villa Bianca, R., ... Calignano, A. (2013). N-Palmitoylethanolamide protects the kidney from hypertensive injury in spontaneously hypertensive rats via inhibition of oxidative stress. *Pharmacol Res, 76*, 67-76. doi:10.1016/j.phrs.2013.07.007

Roncati, L., Lusenti, B., Pellati, F., & Corsi, L. (2021). Micronized / ultramicronized palmitoylethanolamide (PEA) as natural neuroprotector against COVID-19 inflammation. *Prostaglandins Other Lipid Mediat, 154*, 106540. Doi:10.1016/j.prostaglandins.2021.106540

Ruhaak, L., Felth, J., Karlsson, P., Rafter, J/., Verpoorte, R., & Bohlin, L. (2011). Evaluation of the cyclooxygenase inhibiting effects of six major cannabinoids isolated from Cannabis sativa. *Biol Pharm Bull, 34*(5), 774-8. doi:10.1248/bpb.34.774

Russo, E. (2008). Cannabinoids in the management of difficult to treat pain. *Ther Clin Risk Manag, 4*(1), 245-59. doi:10.2147/tcrm.s1928

Russo, E. (2008). Clinical endocannabinoid deficiency (CECD): can this concept explain therapeutic benefits of cannabis in migraine, fibromyalgia, irritable bowel syndrome and other treatment-resistant conditions? *Neuro Endocrinol Lett, 29*(2), 192-200.

Schicho, R., & Storr, M. (2014). Cannabis finds its way into treatment of Crohn's disease. *Pharmacology, 93*(1-2), 1-3. doi:10.1159/000356512

Sheriff, T., Lin, M., Dubin, D., & Khorasani, H. (2020). The potential role of cannabinoids in dermatology. *J Dermatolog Treat, 31*(8), 839-845. doi:10.1080/09546634.2019.1675854

Skaper, S., Facci, L., Barbierato, M., Zusso, M., Bruschetta, G., Impellizzeri, D., ... Giusti, P. (2015). N-Palmitoylethanolamine and neuroinflammation: A novel therapeutic strategy of resolution. *Mol Neurobiol, 52*(2), 1034-42. doi:10.1007/s12035-015-9253-8

Ständer, S., Reinhardt, H., & Luger, T. (2006). [Topical cannabinoid agonists. An effective new possibility for treating chronic pruritus]. [Article in German] *Hautarzt, 57*(9), 801-7. doi:10.1007/s00105-006-1180-1

Stanley, C., Hind, W., & O'Sullivan, S. (2013). Is the cardiovascular system a therapeutic target for cannabidiol? *Br J Clin Pharmacol, 75*(2), 313-22. doi:10.1111/j.1365-2125.2012.04351.x

Steels, E., Venkatesh, R., Steels, E., Vitetta, G., Vitetta, L. (2019). A double-blind randomized placebo-controlled study assessing safety, tolerability and efficacy of palmitoylethanolamide for symptoms of knee osteoarthritis. *Inflammopharmacology, 27*(3), 475-485. doi:10.1007/s10787-019-00582-9

Tagne, A., Pacchetti, B., Sodergren, M., Cosentino, M., & Marino, F. (2020). Cannabidiol for viral diseases: Hype or hope? *Cannabis Cannabinoid Res, 5*(2), 121-131. doi: 10.1089/can.2019.0060

Vuolo, F., Petronilho, F., Sonai, B., Ritter, C., Hallak, J., Zuardi, A., ... Dal-Piozzol, F. (2015). Evaluation of serum cytokines levels and the role of cannabidiol treatment in animal model of asthma. *Mediators Inflamm*, 38670. doi:10.1155/2015/538670

Wassmann, C., Højrup, P., & Klitgaard, J. (2020). Cannabidiol is an effective helper compound in combination with bacitracin to kill Gram-positive bacteria. *Sci Rep, 10*(1), 4112. doi:10.1038/s41598-020-60952-0

Xiong, W., Cui, T., Cheng, K., Yang, F., Chen, S., Willenbring, D., ... Zhang, L. (2012). Cannabinoids suppress inflammatory and neuropathic pain by targeting α3 glycine receptors. *J Exp Med, 209*(6), 1121-34. doi:10.1084/jem.20120242

14. Immune Conditions

Angelina, A., Pérez-Diego, M., López-Abente, J., & Palomares, O. (2020). The role of cannabinoids in allergic diseases: Collegium internationale allergologicum (CIA) update. *Int Arch Allergy Immunol, 181*(8), 565-584. doi:10.1159/000508989

Antonucci, N., Cirillo, A., & Siniscalco, D. (2015). Beneficial effects of palmitoylethanolamide on expressive language, cognition, and behaviors in autism: A report of two cases. *Case Rep Psychiatry, 2015*, 325061. doi:10.1155/2015/325061

Artukoglu, B., Beyer, C., Zuloff-Shani, A., Brener, E., & Bloch, M. (2017). Efficacy of palmitoylethanolamide for pain: A meta-analysis. *Pain Physician, 20*(5), 353-362.

De Filippis, D., Negro, L., Vaia, M., Cinelli, M., & Iuvone, T. (2013). New insights in mast cell modulation by palmitoylethanolamide. *CNS Neurol Disord Drug Targets, 12*(1), 78-83. doi:10.2174/1871527311312010013

Dudášová, A., Keir, S., Parsons, M., Molleman, A., & Page, C. (2013). The effects of cannabidiol on the antigen-induced contraction of airways smooth muscle in the guinea-pig. *Pulm Pharmacol Ther, 26*(3), 373-9. doi:10.1016/j.pupt.2013.02.002

Facci, L., Dal Toso, R., Romanello, S., Buriani, A., Skaper, S., & Leon, A. (1995). Mast cells express a peripheral cannabinoid receptor with differential sensitivity to anandamide and palmitoylethanolamide. *Proc Natl Acad Sci U S A, 92*(8), 3376-80. doi:10.1073/pnas.92.8.3376

Kytikova, O., Novgorodtseva, T., Antonyuk, M., Denisenko, Y., & Gvozdenko, T. (2019). Molecular targets of fatty acid ethanolamides in asthma. *Medicina (Kaunas), 55*(4), 87. doi:10.3390/medicina55040087

Vaia, M., Petrosino, S., De Filippis, D., Negro, L., Guarino, A., Carnuccio, R., … Iuvone, T. (2016). Palmitoylethanolamide reduces inflammation and itch in a mouse model of contact allergic dermatitis. *Eur J Pharmacol, 791*, 669-674. doi:10.1016/j.ejphar.2016.10 .005

15. Metabolic Conditions

Esposito, K., & Giugliano, D. (2004). The metabolic syndrome and inflammation: association or causation. *Nutr Metab Cardiovasc Dis, 14*(5), 228-32. doi:10.1016/s0939-4753(04)80048-6

Esser, N., Paquot, N., & Scheen, A. (2015). Anti-inflammatory agents to treat or prevent type 2 diabetes, metabolic syndrome and cardiovascular disease. *Expert Opin Investig Drugs,* *24*(3), 283-307. doi:10.1517/13543784.2015.974804

Griffiths, E., & Rutter, G. (2009). Mitochondrial calcium as a key regulator of mitochondrial ATP production in mammalian cells. *Biochim Biophys Acta, 1787*(11), 1324-33. doi:10.1016/j.bbabio.2009.01.019

Jadoon, K., Ratcliffe, S., Barrett, D., Thomas, E., Stott, C., Bell, J., … Tan, G. (2016). Efficacy and safety of cannabidiol and tetrahydrocannabivarin on glycemic and lipid parameters in patients with type 2 diabetes: A randomized, double-blind, placebo-controlled, parallel group pilot study. *Diabetes Care, 39*(10), 1777-86. doi:10.2337/dc16-0650

Kim, D., Kim, W., Kwak, M., Chung, G., Yim, J., & Ahmed, A. (2017). Inverse association of marijuana use with non-alcoholic fatty liver disease among adults in the United States. *PLoS One, 12*(10), e0186702. doi:10.1371/journal.pone.0186702

Parray, H., & Yun, J. (2016). Cannabidiol promotes browning in 3T3-L1 adipocytes. *Mol Cell Biochem, 416*(1-2), 131-9. doi:10.1007/s11010-016-2702-5

Reddy, P., Lent-Schochet, D., Ramakrishnan, N., McLaughlin, M., & Jialal, I. (2019). Metabolic syndrome is an inflammatory disorder: A conspiracy between adipose tissue and phagocytes. *Clin Chim Acta,* *496,* 35-44. doi:10.1016/j.cca.2019.06.019

Rossi, F., Punzo, F., Umano, G., Argenziano, M., & Del Giudice, E. (2018). Role of cannabinoids in obesity. *Int J Mol Sci, 19(*9), 2690. doi:10.3390/ijms19092690

Ryan, D., Drysdale, A., Lafourcade, C., Pertwee, R., & Platt, B. (2009). Cannabidiol targets mitochondria to regulate intracellular Ca2+ levels. *J Neurosci, 29*(7), 2053-63. doi:10.1523/JNEUROSCI.4212-08.2009

Schifilliti, C., Cucinotta, L., Fedele, V., Ingegnosi, C., Luca, S., & Leotta, C. (2014). Micronized palmitoylethanolamide reduces the symptoms of neuropathic pain in diabetic patients. *Pain Res Treat, 2014,* 849623. doi:10.1155/2014/849623

Spanagel, R., & Bilbao,A. (2021). Approved cannabinoids for medical purposes - comparative systematic review and meta-analysis for sleep and appetite. *Neuropharmacology, 196,* 108680. doi:10. 1016/j.neuropharm.2021.108680

Waterreus, A., Di Prinzio, A., Watts, G., Castle, D., Galletly, D & Morgan, V. (2016). Metabolic syndrome in people with a psychotic illness: Is cannabis protective? *Psychol Med, 46*(8), 1651-62. doi:10. 1017/S0033291715002883

Welty, F., Alfaddagh, A., & Elajami, T. (2016). Targeting inflammation in metabolic syndrome. *Transl Res, 167*(1), 257-80. doi:10.1016/j.trsl.2015.06.017

16. Neurological Conditions

Aghaei, I., Rostampour, M., Shabani, M., Naderi, N., Motamedi, F., Babaei, P., & Khakpour-Taleghani, B. (2015). Palmitoylethanolamide attenuates PTZ-induced seizures through CB1 and CB2 receptors. *Epilepsy Res, 117,* 23-8. doi:10.1016/j.eplepsyres.2015.08.010

Akinyemi, E., Randhawa, G., Longoria, V., & Zeine, R. (2020). Medical marijuana effects in movement disorders, focus on Huntington disease: A literature review. *J Pharm Pharm Sci, 23*. doi:10.18433/jpps30967

Assogna, M., Casula, E., Borghi, I., Bonnì, S., Samà, D., Motta, C., ... Koch, G. (2020). Effects of palmitoylethanolamide combined with luteoline on frontal lobe functions, high frequency oscillations, and GABAergic transmission in patients with frontotemporal dementia. *J Alzheimers Dis, 76*(4), 1297-1308. doi: 10.3233/JAD-200426

Baron, E. (2018). Medicinal properties of cannabinoids, terpenes, and flavonoids in cannabis, and benefits in migraine, headache, and pain: An update on current evidence and cannabis science. *Headache, 58*(7), 1139-1186. doi:10.1111/head.13345

Baron, E., Lucas, P., Eades, J., & Hogue, O. (2018). Patterns of medicinal cannabis use, strain analysis, and substitution effect among patients with migraine, headache, arthritis, and chronic pain in a medicinal cannabis cohort. *J Headache Pain, 19*(1), 37. doi:10 .1186/s10194-018-0862-2

Beggiato, S., Tomasini, M., & Ferraro, L. (2019). Palmitoylethanolamide (PEA) as a potential therapeutic agent in Alzheimer's disease. *Front Pharmacol, 10*, 821. doi:10.3389/fphar.2019.00821

Bénard, G., Massa, F., Puente, N., Lourenço, J., Bellocchio, L., Soria-Gómez, E., … Marsicano, G. (2012). Mitochondrial CB$_1$ receptors regulate neuronal energy metabolism. *Nat Neurosci, 15*(4), 558-64. doi:10.1038/nn.3053

Boychuk, D., Goddard, G., Mauro, G., & Orellana, M. (2015). The effectiveness of cannabinoids in the management of chronic non-malignant neuropathic pain: A systematic review. *J Oral Facial Pain Headache, 29*(1), 7-14. doi:10.11607/ofph.1274

Brotini, S., Schievano, C., & Guidi, L. (2017). Ultramicronized palmitoylethanolamide: An efficacious adjuvant therapy for Parkinson's disease. *CNS Neurol Disord Drug Targets, 16*(6), 705-713. doi:10.2174/1871527316666170321124949

Carlsen, E., Falk, S., Skupio, U., Robin, L., Zottola, A., Marsicano, G., & Perrier, J. (2021). Spinal astroglial cannabinoid receptors control pathological tremor. *Nat Neurosci, 24*(5), 658-666. doi:10.1038/s41593-021-00818-4

Chagas, M., Zuardi, A., Tumas, V., Pena-Pereira, M., Sobreira, E., Bergamaschi, M., … Crippa, J. (2014). Effects of cannabidiol in the treatment of patients with Parkinson's disease: An exploratory double-blind trial. *J Psychopharmacol, 28*(11), 1088-98. doi:10.1177/0269881114550355

Chagas, M., Eckeli, A., Zuardi, A., Pena-Pereira, M., Sobreira-Neto, M., Sobreira, E., … Crippa, J. (2014). Cannabidiol can improve complex sleep-related behaviours associated with rapid eye movement sleep behaviour disorder in Parkinson's disease patients: A case series. *J Clin Pharm Ther, 39*(5), 564-6. doi:10.1111/jcpt.12179

Chirchiglia, D., Cione, E., Caroleo, M., Wang, M., Di Mizio, G., Faedda, N., … Gallelli, L. (2018). Effects of add-on ultramicronized N-palmitol ethanol amide in patients suffering of migraine with aura: A pilot study. *Front Neurol, 9*, 674. doi:10.3389/fneur.2018.00674

Crippa, J., Hallak, J., Zuardi, A., Francisco S., Guimarães, F., Tumas, V., & Dos Santos, R. (2019). Is cannabidiol the ideal drug to treat non-motor Parkinson's disease symptoms? *Eur Arch Psychiatry Clin Neurosci, 269*(1), 121-133. doi:10.1007/s00406-019-00982-6

Crupi, R., Impellizzeri, D., Cordaro, M., Siracusa, R., Casili, G., Evangelista, M., & Cuzzocrea, S. (2018). N-palmitoylethanolamide prevents Parkinsonian phenotypes in aged mice. *Mol Neurobiol, 55*(11), 8455-8472. doi:10.1007/s12035-018-0959-2

de Faria, S., Fabrício, D., Tumas, V., Castro, P., Ponti, M., Hallak, J., … Chagas, M. (2020). Effects of acute cannabidiol administration on anxiety and tremors induced by a simulated public speaking test in patients with Parkinson's disease. *J Psychopharmacol, 34*(2), 189-196. doi:10.1177/0269881119895536

Esposito, E., Impellizzeri, D., Mazzon, E., Paterniti, I., & Cuzzocrea, S. (2012). Neuroprotective activities of palmitoylethanolamide in an animal model of Parkinson's disease. *PLoS One, 7*(8), e41880. doi:10.1371/journal.pone.0041880

Fernández-Ruiz, J., Sagredo, O., Pazos, M., García, C., Pertwee, R., Mechoulam, R., & Martínez-Orgado, J. (2013). Cannabidiol for neurodegenerative disorders: Important new clinical applications for this phytocannabinoid? *Br J Clin Pharmacol, 75*(2), 323-33. doi:10.1111/j.1365-2125.2012.04341.x

Fiani, B., Sarhadi, K., Soula, M., Zafar, A., & Quadri, S. (2020). Current application of cannabidiol (CBD) in the management and treatment of neurological disorders. *Neurol Sci, 41*(11), 3085-3098. doi:10.1007/s10072-020-04514-2

Gagliano, C., Ortisi, E., Pulvirenti, L., Reibaldi, M., Scollo, D., Amato, R., ... Longo, A. (2011). Ocular hypotensive effect of oral palmitoyl-ethanolamide: A clinical trial. *Invest Ophthalmol Vis Sci, 52*(9), 6096-100. doi:10.1167/iovs.10-7057

Gray, R., & Whalley, B. (2020). The proposed mechanisms of action of CBD in epilepsy. *Epileptic Disord, 22*(S1), 10-15. doi:10.1684/epd.2020.1135

Hoekstra, C., Rynja, S., van Zanten, G., & Rovers, M. (2011). Anticonvulsants for tinnitus. *Cochrane Database Syst Rev, 2011*(7), CD007960. doi:10.1002/14651858.CD007960.pub2

Hounie, A., & Vasques, M. (2019). Neurological improvement with medical cannabis in a progressive supranuclear palsy patient: A case report. *Med Cannabis Cannabinoids, 2*(2), 65-68. doi:10.1159/000503864

Hriday Patra, P., Barker-Haliski, M., White, H., Whalley, B., Glyn, S., Sandhu, H., ... McNeish, A. (2019). Cannabidiol reduces seizures and associated behavioral comorbidities in a range of animal seizure and epilepsy models. *Epilepsia, 60*(2), 303-314. doi:10.1111/epi.14629

Iannotti, F., Hill, C., Leo, A., Alhusaini, A., Soubrane, C., Mazzarella, E., ... Stephens, G. (2014). Nonpsychotropic plant cannabinoids, cannabidivarin (CBDV) and cannabidiol (CBD), activate and desensitize transient receptor potential vanilloid 1 (TRPV1) channels in vitro: potential for the treatment of neuronal hyperexcitability. *ACS Chem Neurosci, 5*(11), 1131-41. doi:10.1021/cn5000524

Jakubovski, E., & Müller-Vahl, K. (2017). Speechlessness in Gilles de la Tourette syndrome: Cannabis-based medicines improve severe vocal blocking tics in two patients. *Int J Mol Sci, 18*(8), 1739. doi:10.3390/ijms18081739

Jones, N., Hill, A., Smith, I., Bevan, S., Williams, C., Whalley, B., & Stephens, G. (2010). Cannabidiol displays antiepileptiform and antiseizure properties in vitro and in vivo. *J Pharmacol Exp Ther, 332*(2), 569-77. doi:10.1124/jpet.109.159145

Kim, S., Yang, J., Kim, K., Kim, J., & Yook, T. (2019). A review on studies of marijuana for Alzheimer's disease - focusing on CBD, THC. *J Pharmacopuncture, 22*(4), 225-230. doi:10.3831/KPI.2019.22.030

Lambert, D., Vandevoorde, S., Diependaele, G., Govaerts, S., & Robert, A. (2001). Anticonvulsant activity of N-palmitoylethanolamide, a putative endocannabinoid, in mice. *Epilepsia, 42*(3), 321-7. doi:10.1046/j.1528-1157.2001.41499.x

Leimuranta, P., Khiroug, L., & Giniatullin, R. (2018). Emerging role of (endo)cannabinoids in migraine. *Front Pharmacol, 9*, 420. doi:10.3389/fphar.2018.00420

Lochte, B., Beletsky, A., Samuel, N., & Grant, I. (2017). The use of cannabis for headache disorders. *Cannabis Cannabinoid Res, 2*(1), 61-71. doi:10.1089/can.2016.0033

Meng, H., Johnston, B., Englesakis, M., Moulin, D., & Bhatia, A. (2017). Selective cannabinoids for chronic neuropathic pain: A systematic review and meta-analysis. *Anesth Analg, 125*(5), 1638-1652. doi: 10.1213/ANE.0000000000002110

Papetti, L., Sforza, G., Tullo, G., di Loro, P., Moavero, R., Ursitti, F., ... Valeriani, M. (2020). Tolerability of palmitoylethanolamide in a pediatric population suffering from migraine: A pilot study. *Pain Res Manag*, 3938640. doi:10.1155/2020/3938640

Peres, F., Lima, A., Hallak, J., Crippa, J., Silva, R., & Abílio, V. (2018). Cannabidiol as a promising strategy to treat and prevent movement disorders? *Front Pharmacol, 9*, 482. doi:10.3389/fphar.2018.00482

Perin, P., Tagne, A., Enrico, P., Marino, F., Cosentino, M., Pizzala, R., & Boselli, C. (2020). Cannabinoids, inner ear, hearing, and tinnitus: A neuroimmunological perspective. *Front Neurol, 11*, 505995. doi:10.3389/fneur.2020.505995

Post, J., Loch, S., Lerner, R., Remmers, F., Lomazzo, E., Lutz, B., & Bindila, L. (2018). Antiepileptogenic effect of subchronic palmitoylethanolamide treatment in a mouse model of acute epilepsy. *Front Mol Neurosci, 11*, 67. doi:10.3389/fnmol.2018.00067

Reiman, A., Welty, M., & Solomon, P. (2017). Cannabis as a substitute for opioid-based pain medication: Patient self-report. *Cannabis Cannabinoid Res, 2*(1), 160-166. doi:10.1089/can.2017.0012

Rossi, G., Scudeller, L., Lumini, C., Bettio, F., Picasso, E., Ruberto, G., ... Bianchi, E. (2020). Effect of palmitoylethanolamide on inner retinal function in glaucoma: A randomized, single blind, crossover, clinical trial by pattern-electroretinogram. *Sci Rep, 10*(1), 10468. doi:10.1038/s41598-020-67527-z

Ryan, D., Drysdale, A., Lafourcade, C., Pertwee, R., & Platt, B. (2009). Cannabidiol targets mitochondria to regulate intracellular Ca2+ levels. *J Neurosci, 29*(7), 2053-63. doi:10.1523/JNEUROSCI.4212-08.2009

Santos de Alencar, S., Crippa, J., Brito, M., Pimentel, A., Hallak, J., & Tumas, V. (2021) .A single oral dose of cannabidiol did not reduce upper limb tremor in patients with essential tremor. *Parkinsonism Relat Disord, 83*, 37-40. doi:10.1016/j.parkreldis.2021.01.001

Sarchielli, P., Pini, L., Coppola, F., Rossi, C., Baldi, A., Mancini, M., & Calabresi, P. (2007). Endocannabinoids in chronic migraine: CSF findings suggest a system failure. *Neuropsychopharmacology, 32*(6), 1384-90. doi:10.1038/sj.npp.1301246

Scuderi, C., Bronzuoli, M., Facchinetti, R., Pace, L., Ferraro, L., Broad, K., … Cassano, T. (2018). Ultramicronized palmitoylethanolamide rescues learning and memory impairments in a triple transgenic mouse model of Alzheimer's disease by exerting anti-inflammatory and neuroprotective effects. *Transl Psychiatry, 8*(1), 32. doi:10.1038/s41398-017-0076-4

Scuderi, C., Steardo, L., & Esposito, G. (2014). Cannabidiol promotes amyloid precursor protein ubiquitination and reduction of beta amyloid expression in SHSY5YAPP+ cells through PPARγ involvement. *Phytother Res, 28*(7), 1007-13. doi:10.1002/ptr.5095

Sheerin, A., Zhang, X., Saucier, D., & Corcoran, M. (2004). Selective antiepileptic effects of N-palmitoylethanolamide, a putative endocannabinoid. *Epilepsia, 45*(10), 1184-8. doi:10.1111/j.0013-9580. 2004.16604.x

Silvestro, S., Mammana, S., Cavalli, E., Bramanti, P., & Mazzon, E. (2019). Use of cannabidiol in the treatment of epilepsy: Efficacy and security in clinical trials. *Molecules, 24*(8), 1459. doi:10.3390/molecules 24081459

Smith, P., & Zheng, Y. (2016). Cannabinoids, cannabinoid receptors and tinnitus. *Hear Res, 332,* 210-216. doi:10.1016/j.heares.2015.09.014

Stockings, E., Campbell, G., Hall, W., Nielsen, S., Zagic, D., Rahman, R., ... Degenhardt, L. (2018). Cannabis and cannabinoids for the treatment of people with chronic noncancer pain conditions: A systematic review and meta-analysis of controlled and observational studies. *Pain, 159*(10), 1932-1954. Doi:10.1097/j.pain.0000000000001293

Strobbe, E., Cellini, M., & Campos, E. (2013). Effectiveness of palmitoylethanolamide on endothelial dysfunction in ocular hypertensive patients: A randomized, placebo-controlled cross over study. *Invest Ophthalmol Vis Sci, 54*(2), 968-73. doi:10.1167/iovs.12-10899

Thaler, A., Arad, S., Bar-Lev Schleider, L., Knaani, J., Taichman, T., Giladi, N., & Gurevich, T. (2019). Single center experience with medical cannabis in Gilles de la Tourette syndrome. *Parkinsonism Relat Disord, 61*, 211-213. doi:10.1016/j.parkreldis.2018.10.004

Tomida, I., Azuara-Blanco, A., House, H., Flint, M., Pertwee, R., & Robson, P. (2006). Effect of sublingual application of cannabinoids on intraocular pressure: A pilot study. *J Glaucoma, 15(*5), 349-53. doi:10.1097/01.ijg.0000212260.04488.60

Tomida, I., Pertwee, R., & Azuara-Blanco, A. (2004). Cannabinoids and glaucoma. *Br J Ophthalmol, 88*(5), 708-13. doi:10.1136/bjo.2003.032250

Zheng, Y., Reid, P., & Smith, P. (2015). Cannabinoid CB1 receptor agonists do not decrease, but may increase acoustic trauma-induced tinnitus in rats. *Front Neurol, 6*, 60. doi:10.3389/fneur.2015.00060

Zuardi, A., Crippa, J., Hallak, J., Pinto, J., Chagas, M., Rodrigues, G.,.... Tumas, V. (2009). Cannabidiol for the treatment of psychosis in Parkinson's disease. *J Psychopharmacol, 23*(8), 979-83. doi:10.1177/0269881 108096519

17. Behavioural Conditions

Andries, A., Frystyk, J., Flyvbjerg, A., & Støving, R. (2014). Dronabinol in severe, enduring anorexia nervosa: a randomized controlled trial. *Int J Eat Disord, 47*(1), 18-23. doi:10.1002/eat.22173

Antonucci, N., Cirillo, A., & Siniscalco, D. (2015). Beneficial effects of palmitoylethanolamide on expressive language, cognition, and behaviors in autism: A report of two cases. *Case Rep Psychiatry, 2015,* 325061. doi:10.1155/2015/325061

Aran, A., Cassuto, H., Lubotzky, A., Wattad, N., & Hazan, E. (2019). Brief report: Cannabidiol-rich cannabis in children with autism spectrum disorder and severe behavioral problems-a retrospective feasibility study. *J Autism Dev Disord, 49*(3), 1284-1288. doi:10.1007/s10803-018-3808-2

Aran, A., Harel, M., Cassuto, H., Polyansky, L., Schnapp, A., Wattad, N., ... Castellanos, F. (2021). Cannabinoid treatment for autism: A proof-of-concept randomized trial. *Mol Autism,* *12*(1), 6. doi:10.1186/s13229-021-00420-2

Aran, A., Eylon, M., Harel, M., Polianski, L., Nemirovski, A., Tepper, S., ... Tam, W. (2019). Lower circulating endocannabinoid levels in children with autism spectrum disorder. *Mol Autism, 10,* 2. doi:10.1186/s13229-019-0256-6

Barchel, D., Stolar, O., De-Haan, T., Ziv-Baran, T., Saban, N., Fuchs, D., ... Berkovitch, M. (2019). Oral cannabidiol use in children with autism spectrum disorder to treat related symptoms and comorbidities. *Front Pharmacol, 9,* 1521. doi:10.3389/fphar. 2018.01521

Bar-Lev Schleider, L., Mechoulam, R., Saban, N., Meiri, G., & Novack, V. (2019). Real life experience of medical cannabis treatment in autism: Analysis of safety and efficacy. *Sci Rep, 9*(1), 200. doi:10.1038/ s41598-018-37570-y

Bitencourt, R & Takahashi, R. (2018). Cannabidiol as a Therapeutic alternative for post-traumatic stress disorder: From bench research to confirmation in human trials. *Front Neurosci, 12,* 502. doi:10.3389/fnins. 2018.00502

Blessing, E., Steenkamp, M., Manzanares, J., & Marmar, C. (2015). Cannabidiol as a potential treatment for anxiety disorders. *Neurotherapeutics*, *12*(4), 825-36. doi:10.1007/s13311-015-0387-1

Blinder, B., Cumella, E., & Sanathara, V. (2006). Psychiatric comorbidities of female inpatients with eating disorders. *Psychosom Med, 68*(3), 454-62. doi:10.1097/01.psy.0000221254.77675.f5

Collu, R., Scherma, M., Piscitelli, F., Giunti, E., Satta, V., Castelli, M., ... Fadda, P. (2019). Impaired brain endocannabinoid tone in the activity-based model of anorexia nervosa. *Int J Eat Disord, 52*(11), 1251-1262. doi:10.1002/eat.23157

Crippa, J., Guimarães, F., Campos, A., & Zuardi, A. (2018). Translational investigation of the therapeutic potential of cannabidiol (CBD): Toward a new age. *Front Immunol, 9*, 2009. doi:10.3389/fimmu.2018 .02009

Cristiano, C., Pirozzi, C., Coretti, L., Cavaliere, G., Lama, A., Russo, R., ... Raso, G. (2018). Palmitoylethanolamide counteracts autistic-like behaviours in BTBR T+tf/J mice: Contribution of central and peripheral mechanisms. *Brain Behav Immun, 74*, 166-175. doi:10.1016/j.bbi.2018.09.003

Davies, C., & Bhattacharyya, S. (2019). Cannabidiol as a potential treatment for psychosis. *Ther Adv*

Psychopharmacol, 9, 2045125319881916. doi:10.1177 /2045125319881916

De Gregorio, D., Manchia, M., Carpiniello, B., Valtorta, F., Nobile, M., Gobbi, G., & Comai, S. (2019). Role of palmitoylethanolamide (PEA) in depression: Translational evidence: Special Section on "Translational and Neuroscience Studies in Affective Disorders". *J Affect Disord, 255,* S0165-0327(18)31599-4. doi:10.1016/j.jad.2018.10.117

De Marchi, N., De Petrocellis, L., Orlando, P., Daniele, F., Fezza, F., & Di Marzo, V. (2003). Endocannabinoid signalling in the blood of patients with schizophrenia. *Lipids Health Dis, 2,* 5. doi:10.1186/1476-511X-2-5

Elms, L., Shannon, S., Hughes, S., & Lewis, N. (2019). Cannabidiol in the treatment of post-traumatic stress disorder: A case series. *J Altern Complement Med, 25*(4), 392-397. doi:10.1089/acm.2018.0437

Evangelista, M., Cilli, De Vitis, R., Militerno, A., & Fanfani,F. (2018). Ultramicronized palmitoylethanolamide effects on sleep-wake rhythm and neuropathic pain phenotypes in patients with carpal tunnel syndrome: An open-label, randomized controlled study. *CNS Neurol Disord Drug Targets, 17*(4), 291-298. doi:10.2174/1871527317666180420143830

Fleury-Teixeira, P., Caixeta, F., Ramires da Silva, L., Brasil-Neto, J., & Malcher-Lopes, R. (2019). Effects of CBD-enriched *Cannabis sativa* extract on autism spectrum disorder symptoms: An observational study of 18 participants undergoing compassionate use. *Front Neurol, 10*, 1145. doi:10.3389/fneur.2019.01145

Ghazizadeh-Hashemi, M., Ghajar, A., Shalbafan, M., Ghazizadeh-Hashemi, F., Afarideh, M., Malekpour, F., ... Akhondzadeh, S. (2018). Palmitoylethanolamide as adjunctive therapy in major depressive disorder: A double-blind, randomized and placebo-controlled trial. *J Affect Disord, 232*, 127-133. doi:10.1016/j.jad.2018.02.057

Gorzalka, B., & Hill, M. (2009). Integration of endocannabinoid signaling into the neural network regulating stress-induced activation of the hypothalamic-pituitary-adrenal axis. *Curr Top Behav Neurosci, 1*, 289-306. doi:10.1007/978-3-540-88955 7_12

Hill, M., Kumar, S., Filipski, S., Iverson, M., Stuhr, K., Keith, J., ... McEwen, B. (2013). Disruption of fatty acid amide hydrolase activity prevents the effects of chronic stress on anxiety and amygdala microstructure. *Mol Psychiatry, 18*(10), 1125-35. doi:10.1038/mp.2012.90

Hillard, C. (2014). Stress regulates endocannabinoid-CB1 receptor signaling. *Semin Immunol, 26*(5), 380-8. doi:10.1016/j.smim.2014.04.001

Ho, B., Wassink, T., Ziebell, S., Andreasen, N. (2011). Cannabinoid receptor 1 gene polymorphisms and marijuana misuse interactions on white matter and cognitive deficits in schizophrenia. *Schizophr Res, 128*(1-3), 66-75. doi:10.1016/j.schres.2011.02.021

Khalaj, M., Saghazadeh, A., Shirazi, E., Shalbafan, M., Alavi, K., Shooshtari, M., ... Akhondzadeh, S. (2018). Palmitoylethanolamide as adjunctive therapy for autism: Efficacy and safety results from a randomized controlled trial. *J Psychiatr Res, 103*, 104-111. doi:10.1016/j.jpsychires.2018.04.022

Lake, J. (2014). A review of select CAM modalities for the prevention and treatment of PTSD. *Psychiatric Times, 31*(7), 29

Leweke, F., Piomelli, D., Pahlisch, F., Muhl, D.,Gerth, C., Hoyer, C., ... Koethe, D. (2012). Cannabidiol enhances anandamide signaling and alleviates psychotic symptoms of schizophrenia. *Transl Psychiatry, 2*(3), e94. doi:10.1038/tp.2012.15

Locci, A., & Pinna, G. (2019). Stimulation of peroxisome proliferator-activated receptor-α by N-palmitoylethanolamine engages allopregnanolone biosynthesis to modulate emotional behavior. *Biol Psychiatry, 85*(12), 1036-1045. doi:10.1016/j.biopsych .2019.02.006

Lutz, B., Marsicano, G., Maldonado, R., & Hillard, C. (2015). The endocannabinoid system in guarding against fear, anxiety and stress. *Nat Rev Neurosci, 16*(12), 705-18. doi:10.1038/nrn4036

Monteleone, A., Di Marzo, V., Aveta, T., Piscitelli, F., Dalle Grave, R., Scognamiglio, P., ... Maj, M. (2015). Deranged endocannabinoid responses to hedonic eating in underweight and recently weight-restored patients with anorexia nervosa. *Am J Clin Nutr, 101*(2), 262-9. doi:10.3945/ajcn.114.096164

Monteleone, P., Bifulco, M., Di Filippo, C., Gazzerro, P., Canestrelli, B., Monteleone, F., ... Maj, M. (2009). Association of CNR1 and FAAH endocannabinoid gene polymorphisms with anorexia nervosa and bulimia nervosa: Evidence for synergistic effects. *Genes Brain Behav, 8*(7), 728-32. doi:10.1111/j.1601-183X.2009 .00518.x

Murillo-Rodríguez, E. (2008). The role of the CB1 receptor in the regulation of sleep. *Prog Neuropsychopharmacol Biol Psychiatry, 32*(6), 1420-7. doi:10.1016/j.pnpbp.2008.04.008

Radhakrishnan, R., Wilkinson, S., & D'Souza, D. (2014). Gone to pot: A review of the association between cannabis and psychosis. *Front Psychiatry, 5,* 54. doi:10.3389/fpsyt.2014.00054

Rao, A., Ebelt, P., Mallard, A., & Briskey, D. (2021). Palmitoylethanolamide for sleep disturbance: A double-blind, randomised, placebo-controlled interventional study. *Sleep Sci Pract, 5*(1), 12. doi:10.1186/s41606-021-00065-3

Reiman, A., Welty, M., & Solomon, P. (2017). Cannabis as a substitute for opioid-based pain medication: Patient self-report. *Cannabis Cannabinoid Res, 2*(1), 160-166. doi:10.1089/can.2017.0012

Riebe, C., & Wotjak, C. (2011). Endocannabinoids and stress. *Stress, 14*(4), 384-97.doi:10.3109/10253890 .2011.586753

Rosager, E., Møller, C., & Sjögren, M. (2021). Treatment studies with cannabinoids in anorexia nervosa: A systematic review. *Eat Weight Disord, 26*(2), 407-415. doi:10.1007/s40519-020-00891-x

Russo, E., Burnett, A., Hall, B., & Parker, K. (2005). Agonistic properties of cannabidiol at 5-HT1a receptors. *Neurochem Res, 30*(8), 1037-43. doi:10.1007/s11064-005-6978-1

Sabelli, H., Fink, P., Fawcett, J., & Tom, C. (1996). Sustained antidepressant effect of PEA replacement. *J Neuropsychiatry Clin Neurosci, 8*(2), 168-71. doi:10.1176/jnp.8.2.168

Sales, A., Fogaça, M., Sartim, A., Pereira, V., Wegener, G., Guimarães, F., & Joca, S. (2019). Cannabidiol induces rapid and sustained antidepressant-like effects through increased BDNF signaling and synaptogenesis in the prefrontal cortex. *Mol Neurobiol, 56*(2), 1070-1081. doi:10.1007/s12035-018-1143-4

Schier, A., Ribeiro, N., Coutinho, D., Machado, S., Arias-Carrión, O., Crippa, J., …Silva, A. (2014). Antidepressant-like and anxiolytic-like effects of cannabidiol: A chemical compound of Cannabis sativa. *CNS Neurol Disord Drug Targets, 13*(6), 953-60. doi:10.2174/1871527313666140612114838

Schier, A., Ribeiro, N., Silva, A., Hallak, J., Crippa, J., Nardi, N., Zuardi, A. (2012). Cannabidiol, a Cannabis sativa constituent, as an anxiolytic drug. [Article in English, Portuguese] *Braz J Psychiatry, 34* Suppl 1, S104-10. doi:10.1590/s1516-44462012000500008

Scolnick, B. (2018). Treatment of anorexia nervosa with palmitoylethanoamide. *Med Hypotheses, 116*, 54-60. doi:10.1016/j.mehy.2018.04.010

Shannon, S., & Opila-Lehman, J. (2016). Effectiveness of cannabidiol oil for pediatric anxiety and insomnia as part of posttraumatic stress disorder: A case report. *Perm J, 20*(4), 16-005. doi:10.7812/TPP/16-005

Skaper, S., & Facci, L. (2012). Mast cell-glia axis in neuroinflammation and therapeutic potential of the anandamide congener palmitoylethanolamide. *Philos Trans R Soc Lond B Biol Sci, 367*(1607), 3312-25. doi:10.1098/rstb.2011.0391

Skaper, S., Facci, L., & Giusti, P. (2014). Mast cells, glia and neuroinflammation: partners in crime? *Immunology, 141*(3), 314-27. doi:10.1111/imm.12170

Soares, V., & Campos, A. (2017). Evidence for the anti-panic actions of cannabidiol. *Curr Neuropharmacol, 15*(2), 291-299. doi:10.2174/1570159x146661605091 23955

Steels, E., Venkatesh, R., Steels, E., Vitetta, G., & Vitetta, L. (2019). A double-blind randomized placebo-controlled study assessing safety, tolerability and efficacy of palmitoylethanolamide for symptoms of knee osteoarthritis. *Inflammopharmacology, 27*(3), 475-485. doi:10.1007/s10787-019-00582-9

Ujike, H., & Morita, Y. (2004). New perspectives in the studies on endocannabinoid and cannabis: cannabinoid receptors and schizophrenia. *J Pharmacol Sci, 96*(4), 376-81. doi:10.1254/jphs.fmj04003x4

Walsh, J., Maddison, K., Rankin, T., Murray, K., McArdle, N., Ree, M., ... Eastwood, P. (2021). Treating insomnia symptoms with medicinal cannabis: A randomized, crossover trial of the efficacy of a cannabinoid medicine compared with placebo. *Sleep. 44*(11), zsab149. doi:10.1093/sleep/zsab149

Resources

Anorexia Nervosa. The Free Dictionary. Retrieved from https.//medical-dictionary.thefree dictionary.com/anorexia +nervosa

18. Proliferative Conditions

Blázquez, C., Casanova, M., Planas, A., Gómez Del Pulgar, T., Villanueva, C., Fernández-Aceñero, M., ... Guzmán, M. (2003). Inhibition of tumor angiogenesis by cannabinoids. *FASEB J, 17*(3), 529-31. doi: 10.1096/fj.02-0795fje

Casanova, M., Blázquez, C., Martínez-Palacio, J., Villanueva, C., Fernández-Aceñero, M., Huffman, J., ... Guzmán, M. (2003). Inhibition of skin tumor growth and angiogenesis in vivo by activation of cannabinoid receptors. *J Clin Invest,* *111*(1), 43-50. doi: 10.1172/JCI16116

De Petrocellis, L., Melck, D., Palmisano, A., Bisogno, T., Laezza, C., Bifulco, M., & Di Marzo, V. (1998). The endogenous cannabinoid anandamide inhibits human breast cancer cell proliferation. *Proc Natl Acad Sci U S A,* *95*(14), 8375-80. doi: 10.1073/pnas.95.14.8375

De Petrocellis, L., Ligresti, A., Moriello, A., Iappelli, M., Verde, R., Stott, C., ... Di Marzo, V. (2013). Non-THC cannabinoids inhibit prostate carcinoma growth in vitro and in vivo: Pro-apoptotic effects and underlying mechanisms. *Br J Pharmacol,* *168*(1), 79-102. doi: 10.1111/j.1476-5381.2012.02027.x

Deng, L., & Stella, N. (2015). Cannabidiol reduces glioma cells proliferation and viability. *Neuro Oncol,* *17*(Suppl 5), v21. doi: 10.1093/neuonc/nov204.15

Di Marzo, V., Melck, D., Orlando, P., Bisogno, T., Zagoory, O., Bifulco, M., ... De Petrocellis, L. (2001. Palmitoylethanolamide inhibits the expression of fatty acid amide hydrolase and enhances the anti-proliferative effect of anandamide in human breast cancer cells. *Biochem J,* *358*(Pt 1), 249-55. doi: 10.1042/0264-6021:3580249

Hinz, B., & Ramer, R. (2019). Anti-tumour actions of cannabinoids. *Br J Pharmacol, 176*(10), 1384-1394. doi: 10.1111/bph.14426

Hu, G., Ren, G., & Shi, Y. (2011). The putative cannabinoid receptor GPR55 promotes cancer cell proliferation. *Oncogene, 30*(2), 139-41. doi: 10.1038/onc.2010.502

Moreau, M., Ibeh, U., Decosmo, K., Bih, N., Yasmin-Karim, S., Toyang, N., ... Ngwa, W. (2019). Flavonoid derivative of *Cannabis* demonstrates therapeutic potential in preclinical models of metastatic pancreatic cancer. *Front Oncol, 9*, 660. doi: 10.3389/fonc .2019 .00660

Pacher, P. (2013). Towards the use of non-psychoactive cannabinoids for prostate cancer. *Br J Pharmacol, 168*(1), 76-8. doi: 10.1111/j.1476-5381.2012.02121.x

Pan, H., Mukhopadhyay, P., Rajesh, M., Patel, V., Mukhopadhyay, B., Gao, B., ... Pacher, P. (2009). Cannabidiol attenuates cisplatin-induced nephrotoxicity by decreasing oxidative/nitrosative stress, inflammation, and cell death. *J Pharmacol Exp Ther, 328*(3), 708-14. doi: 10.1124/jpet.108.147181

Parker, L., Rock, E., & Limebeer, C. (2011). Regulation of nausea and vomiting by cannabinoids. *Br J*

Pharmacol, 163(7), 1411-22. doi: 10.1111/j.1476-5381.2010.01176.x

Rock, E., Sticht, M., Limebeer, C., & Parker, L. (2016). Cannabinoid regulation of acute and anticipatory nausea. *Cannabis Cannabinoid Res, 1*(1), 113-121. doi: 10.1089/can.2016.0006

Sharafi, G., He, H., & Nikfarjam, M. (2019). Potential use of cannabinoids for the treatment of pancreatic cancer. *J Pancreat Cancer, 5*(1), 1-7. doi: 10.1089/pancan.2018.0019

Shrivastava, A., Kuzontkoski, P., Groopman, J., & Prasad, A. (2011). Cannabidiol induces programmed cell death in breast cancer cells by coordinating the cross-talk between apoptosis and autophagy. *Mol Cancer Ther, 10*(7), 1161-72. doi: 10.1158/1535-7163.MCT-10-1100

Solinas, M., Massi, P., Cantelmo, A., Cattaneo, M., Cammarota, R., Bartolini, D., ... Parolaro, D. (2012). Cannabidiol inhibits angiogenesis by multiple mechanisms. *Br J Pharmacol, 167*(6), 1218-31. doi: 10.1111/j.1476-5381.2012.02050.x

Sulé-Suso, J., Watson, N., van Pittius, D., & Jegannathen, A. (2019). Striking lung cancer response to self-administration of cannabidiol: A case report and literature review. *SAGE Open Med Case Rep, 7*, 2050313X19832160. doi: 10.1177/2050313X19832160

Tudurí, E., Imbernon, M., Hernández-Bautista, R., Tojo, M., Fernø, J., Diéguez, C., & Nogueiras, R. (2017). GPR55: A new promising target for metabolism? *J Mol Endocrinol, 58*(3), R191-R202. doi: 10.1530/JME-16-0253

Ward, S., McAllister, S., Kawamura, R., Murase, R., Neelakantan, H., & Walker, E. (2014) .Cannabidiol inhibits paclitaxel-induced neuropathic pain through 5-HT(1A) receptors without diminishing nervous system function or chemotherapy efficacy. *Br J Pharmacol, 171*(3), 636-45. doi: 10.1111/bph.12439

19. Orphan Diseases

Berger, A., Keefe, J., Winnick, A., Gilbert, E., Eskander, J., Yazdi, C., ... Urtis, I., (2020). Cannabis and cannabidiol (CBD) for the treatment of fibromyalgia. *Best Pract Res Clin Anaesthesiol, 34*(3), 617-631. doi: 10.1016/j.bpa.2020.08.010

Del Giorno, R., Skaper, S., Paladini, A., Varrassi, G., & Coaccioli, S. (2015). Palmitoylethanolamide in fibromyalgia: Results from prospective and retrospective observational studies. *Pain Ther, 4*(2), 169-78. doi: 10.1007/s40122-015-003,8-6

del Río, C., Navarrete, C., Collado, J., Bellido, M., Gómez-Cañas, M., Pazos, M., ... Muñoz, E. (2016). The cannabinoid quinol VCE-004.8 alleviates bleomycin-induced scleroderma and exerts potent antifibrotic effects through peroxisome proliferator-activated receptor-γ and CB2 pathways. *Sci Rep, 6,* 21703. doi: 10.1038/srep21703

Ghorayeb, I. (2020). More evidence of cannabis efficacy in restless legs syndrome. *Sleep Breath, 24*(1), 277-279. doi: 10.1007/s11325-019-01978-1

Hoareau, L., Buyse, M., Festy, F., Ravanan, P., Gonthier, M., Matias, I., ... Roche, R. (2009). Anti-inflammatory effect of palmitoylethanolamide on human adipocytes. *Obesity (Silver Spring), 17*(3), 431-8. doi: 10.1038/oby.2008.591

Impellizzeri, D., Ahmad, A., Bruschetta, G., Di Paola, R., Crupi, R., Paterniti, I., ... Cuzzocrea, S. (2015). The anti-inflammatory effects of palmitoylethanolamide (PEA) on endotoxin-induced uveitis in rats. *Eur J Pharmacol, 761,* 28-35. doi: 10.1016/j.ejphar.2015.04.025

Megelin, T., & Ghorayeb, I. (2017). Cannabis for restless legs syndrome: a report of six patients. *Sleep Med, 36*, 182-183. doi: 10.1016/j.sleep.2017.04.019

Nanchahal, J., Ball, C., Davidson, D., Williams, L., Sones, W., McCann, F., ... Lamb, S., (2018). Anti-tumour necrosis factor therapy for Dupuytren's disease: A randomised dose response proof-of-concept phase 2a clinical trial. *EBioMedicine, 33*, 282-288. doi: 10.1016/j.ebiom.2018.06.022

Petrosino, S., Roberta Verde, R., Vaia, M., Allarà, M., Iuvone, T., & Di Marzo, V. (2018). Anti-inflammatory properties of cannabidiol, a nonpsychotropic cannabinoid, in experimental allergic contact dermatitis. *J Pharmacol Exp Ther, 365*(3), 652-663. doi: 10.1124/jpet.117.244368

Sagy, I., Bar-Lev Schleider, L., Abu-Shakra, M., & Novack, V. (2019). Safety and efficacy of medical cannabis in fibromyalgia. *J Clin Med, 8*(6), 807. doi: 10.3390/jcm8060807

Schweiger, V., Martini, A., Bellamoli, P., Donadello, K., Schievano, C., Balzo, G., ... Polati, E. (2019). Ultramicronized palmitoylethanolamide (um-PEA) as add-on treatment in fibromyalgia syndrome (FMS): Retrospective observational study on 407 patients. *CNS*

Neurol Disord Drug Targets, 18(4), 326-333. doi: 10.2174/1871527318666190227205359

Theoharides, T., Tsilioni, I., & Bawazeer, M. (2019). Mast cells, neuroinflammation and pain in fibromyalgia syndrome. *Front Cell Neurosci, 13*, 353. doi: 10.3389/fncel.2019.00353

20. Women's Health

Armour, M., Sinclair, J., Chalmers, K., & Smith, C. (2019). Self-management strategies amongst Australian women with endometriosis: A national online survey. *BMC Complement Altern Med, 19*(1), 17.doi:10.1186/s12906-019-2431-x

Bilgic, E., Guzel, E., Kose, S., Aydin, M., Karaismailoglu, E., Akar, I., … Korkusuz, P. (2017). Endocannabinoids modulate apoptosis in endometriosis and adenomyosis. *Acta Histochem, 119*(5), 523-532.doi:10.1016/j.acthis.2017.05.005

Escudero-Lara, A., Argerich, J., Cabañero, D., & Maldonado, R. (2020). Disease-modifying effects of natural Δ9-tetrahydrocannabinol in endometriosis-associated pain. *Elife, 9*, e50356. doi:10.7554/eLife .50356

Gorzalka, B., & Dang, S. (2012). Minireview: Endocannabinoids and gonadal hormones: bidirectional interactions in physiology and behavior. *Endocrinology, 153*(3), 1016-24. doi: 10.1210/en.2011-1643

Luschnig, P., & Schicho, R. (2019). Cannabinoids in gynecological diseases. *Med Cannabis Cannabinoids, 2*(1), 14-21. doi:10.1159/000499164

Shams, T., Firwana, B., Habib, F., Alshahrani, A., Alnouh, B., Murad, M., & Ferwana, M. (2014). SSRIs for hot flashes: A systematic review and meta-analysis of randomized trials. *J Gen Intern Med, 29*(1), 204-13. doi: 10.1007/s11606-013-2535-9

Stochino Loi, E., Pontis, A., Cofelice, V., Pirarba, S., Fais, M., Daniilidis, A., ... Angioni, S. (2019). Effect of ultramicronized palmitoylethanolamide and co-micronized palmitoylethanolamide/polydatin on chronic pelvic pain and quality of life in endometriosis patients: An open-label pilot study. *Int J Womens Health, 11*, 443-449. doi: 10.2147/IJWH.S204275

Walker, O., Holloway, A., & Raha, S. (2019). The role of the endocannabinoid system in female reproductive tissues. *J Ovarian Res, 12*(1), 3. doi: 10.1186/s13048-018-0478-9

21. Safety of CBD

Bar-Lev Schleider, L., Mechoulam, R., Lederman, V., Hilou, M., Lencovsky, O., Betzalel, O., ... Novack,V. (2018). Prospective analysis of safety and efficacy of medical cannabis in large unselected population of patients with cancer. *Eur J Intern Med, 49*, 37-43. doi: 10.1016/j.ejim.2018.01.023

World Health Organisation, C*annabidiol (CBD) Critical Review Report.* (2018). https://www.who.int/medicines/access/controlled-substances/CannabidiolCriticalReview.pdf

Cannabinoids associated with negative respiratory health effects in older adults with COPD.(2020). Retrieved from https://scienmag.com/cannabinoids-associated-with-negative-respiratory-health-effects-in-older-adults-with-copd/

Chang, B. (2018). Cannabidiol and serum antiepileptic drug levels: The ABCs of CBD with AEDs. *Epilepsy Curr, 18*(1), 33-34. doi: 10.5698/1535-7597.18.1.33

Chihuri, S., Li, G., & Chen, Q. (2017). Interaction of marijuana and alcohol on fatal motor vehicle crash risk: a case-control study. *Inj Epidemiol, 4*(1), 8. doi: 10.1186/s40621-017-0105-z

Clark, T., Jones, J., Hall, A., Tabner, S., & Kmiec, R. (2018). Theoretical explanation for reduced body mass index and obesity rates in *Cannabis* users. *Cannabis Cannabinoid Res, 3*(1), 259-271. doi: 10.1089/can.2018.0045

Consroe, P., Carlini, E., Zwicker, A., & Lacerda, L. (1979). Interaction of cannabidiol and alcohol in humans. *Psychopharmacology (Berl), 66*(1), 45-50. doi: 10.1007/BF00431988

Deshmukh, N., Gumaste, S., Subah, S., & Bogoda, N. (2021). Palmitoylethanolamide: Prenatal developmental toxicity study in rats. *Int J Toxicol, 40*(2), 161-170. doi: 10.1177/1091581820986073

El Marroun, H., Tiemeier, H., Steegers, E., Jaddoe, V., Hofman, A., Verhulst, F., … Huizink, A. (2009). Intrauterine cannabis exposure affects fetal growth trajectories: the generation R study. *J Am Acad Child Adolesc Psychiatry, 48*(12), 1173-81. doi: 10.1097/CHI.0b013e3181bfa8ee

Ewing, L., Skinner, C., Quick, C., Kennon-McGill, S., McGill, M., Walker, L., … Koturbash, I. (2019). Hepatotoxicity of a cannabidiol-rich cannabis extract in the mouse model. *Molecules, 24*(9), 1694. doi: 10.3390/molecules24091694

Farrimond, J., Whalley, B., & Williams, C. (2012). Cannabinol and cannabidiol exert opposing effects on rat feeding patterns. *Psychopharmacology (Berl), 223*(1), 117-29. doi: 10.1007/s00213-012-2697-x

Feinshtein, V., Erez, O., Ben-Zvi, Z., Erez, N., Eshkoli, T., Sheizaf, B., ... Holcberg, G. (2013). Cannabidiol changes P-gp and BCRP expression in trophoblast cell lines. *PeerJ, 1*, e153. doi: 10.7717/peerj.153

Gable, R. (2006). The toxicity of recreational drugs. *American Scientist, 94,* 206-208

Hartman, R., Brown, T., Milavetz, G., Spurgin, A., Gorelick, D., Gaffney, G., & Huestis, M. (2015). Controlled cannabis vaporizer administration: Blood and plasma cannabinoids with and without alcohol. *Clin Chem, 61*(6), 850-69. doi: 10.1373/clinchem.2015 .238287

Horth, R., Crouch, B., Horowitz, B., Prebish, A., Slawson, M., McNair, J., ... Dunn, A. (2018). Notes from the field: Acute poisonings from a synthetic cannabinoid sold as cannabidiol - Utah, 2017-2018. *MMWR Morb Mortal Wkly Rep, 67*(20), 587-588. doi: 10.15585/mmwr.mm6720a5

Huang, J., Zhang, Z., Tashkin, D., Feng, B., Straif, K., & Hashibe, M. (2015). An epidemiologic review of marijuana and cancer: An update. *Cancer Epidemiol*

Biomarkers Prev, 24(1), 15-31. doi: 10.1158/1055-9965.EPI-14-1026

Hurd, Y., Wang, X., Anderson, V., Beck, O., Minkoff, H., & Dow-Edwards, D. (2005). Marijuana impairs growth in mid-gestation fetuses. *Neurotoxicol Teratol, 27*(2), 221-9. doi: 10.1016/j.ntt.2004.11.002

Iffland, K., & Grotenhermen, F. (2017). An update on safety and side effects of cannabidiol: A review of clinical data and relevant animal studies. *Cannabis Cannabinoid Res, 2*(1), 139-154. doi: 10.1089/can.2016.0034

Jadoon, K., Tan, G., & O'Sullivan, S. (2017). A single dose of cannabidiol reduces blood pressure in healthy volunteers in a randomized crossover study. *JCI Insight, 2*(12), e93760. doi: 10.1172/jci.insight.93760

Jaques, S., Kingsbury, A., Henshcke, P., Chomchai, C., Clews, S., Falconer, J., … Oei, J. (2014). Cannabis, the pregnant woman, and her child: Weeding out the myths. *J Perinatol, 34*(6), 417-24. doi: 10.1038/jp.2013.180

Lachenmeier, D., & Rehm, J. (2015). Comparative risk assessment of alcohol, tobacco, cannabis and other illicit drugs using the margin of exposure approach. *Sci Rep, 5*, 8126. doi: 10.1038/srep08126

Larsen, C., & Shahinas, J. (2020). Dosage, efficacy and safety of cannabidiol administration in adults: A systematic review of human trials. *J Clin Med Res, 12*(3), 129-141. doi: 10.14740/jocmr4090

Nestmann, E. (2016). Safety of micronized palmitoylethanolamide (microPEA): Lack of toxicity and genotoxic potential. *Food Sci Nutr, 5*(2), 292-309. doi: 10.1002/fsn3.392

Park, Y., Linder, D., Pope, J., Flamini, J., Moretz, K., Diamond, M., & Long, S. (2020). Long-term efficacy and safety of cannabidiol (CBD) in children with treatment-resistant epilepsy: Results from a state-based expanded access program. *Epilepsy Behav, 112*, 107474. doi: 10.1016/j.yebeh.2020.107474

Ramer, R., Bublitz, K., Freimuth, N., Merkord, J., Rohde, H., Haustein, M., ... Hinz, B. (2012). Cannabidiol inhibits lung cancer cell invasion and metastasis via intercellular adhesion molecule-1. *FASEB J, 26*(4), 1535-48. doi: 10.1096/fj.11-198184

Sarrafpour, S., Urits, I., Powell, J., Nguyen, D., Callan, J., Orhurhu, V., ... Yazdi, C. (2020).Considerations and implications of cannabidiol use during pregnancy. *Curr Pain Headache Rep, 24*(7), 38. doi: 10.1007/s11916-020-00872-w

Solinas, M., Massi, P., Cantelmo, A., Cattaneo, M., Cammarota, R., Bartolini, D., ... Parolaro, D. (2012). Cannabidiol inhibits angiogenesis by multiple mechanisms. *Br J Pharmacol, 167*(6), 1218-31. doi: 10.1111/j.1476-5381.2012.02050.x

Sultan, S., O'Sullivan, S., & England, T. (2020). The effects of acute and sustained cannabidiol dosing for seven days on the haemodynamics in healthy men: A randomised controlled trial. *Br J Clin Pharmacol, 86*(6), 1125-1138. doi: 10.1111/bcp.14225

Vozoris, N., Pequeno, P., Li, P., Austin, P., Stephenson, A., O'Donnell, D., ... Rochon, P, (2021). Morbidity and mortality associated with prescription cannabinoid drug use in COPD, *Thorax, 76*(1), 29-36. doi: 10.1136/thoraxjnl-2020-215346

Zendulka, O., Dovrtělová, G. Nosková, K., Turjap, M., Šulcová, A., Hanuš, L., & Juřica, J. (2016). Cannabinoids and Cytochrome P450 Interactions. *Curr Drug Metab, 17*(3), 206-26. doi: 10.2174/138 9200217666151210142051

22. How is CBD Used?

Hammell, D., Zhang, L., Ma, F., Abshire, S., McIlwrath, S., Stinchcomb, A., & Westlund, K. (2016).

Transdermal cannabidiol reduces inflammation and pain-related behaviours in a rat model of arthritis. *Eur J Pain, 20*(6), 936-48. doi: 10.1002/ejp.818

Hryhorowicz, S., Walczak, M., Zakerska-Banaszak, O., Słomski, R., & Skrzypczak-Zielińska, M. (2018). Pharmacogenetics of cannabinoids. *Eur J Drug Metab Pharmacokinet, 43*(1), 1–12.doi:10.1007/s13318-017-0416-z

Huestis, M. (2007). Human cannabinoid pharmacokinetics. *Chem Biodivers, 4*(8), 1770-804. doi: 10.1002/cbdv.200790152

Izgelov, D., Domb, A., & Hoffman, A. (2020). The effect of piperine on oral absorption of cannabidiol following acute vs. chronic administration. *Eur J Pharm Sci, 148*, 105313. doi: 10.1016/j.ejps.2020.105313

Kim, J., Li, Y., & Watkins, B. (2011). Endocannabinoid signaling and energy metabolism: A target for dietary intervention. *Nutrition, 27*(6), 624-32. doi: 10.1016/j .nut.2010.11.003

Mannila, J., Järvinen, T., Järvinen, K., & Jarho,P. (2007). Precipitation complexation method produces cannabidiol/beta-cyclodextrin inclusion complex suitable for sublingual administration of cannabidiol. *J Pharm Sci, 96*(2), 312-9. doi: 10.1002/jps.20766

Millar, S., Stone, N., Yates, A., & O'Sullivan, S. (2018). A systematic review on the pharmacokinetics of cannabidiol in humans. *Front Pharmacol, 9*, 1365. doi: 10.3389/fphar.2018.01365

Perucca, E., & Bialer, M. (2020). Critical aspects affecting cannabidiol oral bioavailability and metabolic elimination, and related clinical implications. *CNS Drugs, 34*(8), 795-800. doi: 10.1007/s40263-020-00741-5

Rahimi, A., Faizi, M., Talebi, F., Noorbakhsh, F., Kahrizi, F., & Naderi,N. (2015). Interaction between the protective effects of cannabidiol and palmitoylethanolamide in experimental model of multiple sclerosis in C57BL/6 mice. *Neuroscience, 290*, 279-87. doi: 10.1016/j.neuroscience.2015.01.030

Samara, E., Bialer, M., & Mechoulam, R. (1988). Pharmacokinetics of cannabidiol in dogs. *Drug Metab Dispos, 16*(3), 469-72.

Schicho, R., & Storr, M. (2012). Topical and systemic cannabidiol improves trinitrobenzene sulfonic acid colitis in mice. *Pharmacology, 89*(3-4), 149-55. doi:10.1159/000336871

Tagne, A., Fotio, Y., Lin, L., Squire, E., Ahmed, F., Rashid, T., ... Piomelli, D. (2021). Palmitoylethanolamide and hemp oil extract exert synergistic anti-nociceptive effects in mouse models of acute and chronic pain. *Pharmacol Res, 167,* 105545. doi: 10.1016/j.phrs.2021.105545

Resources

https:// www. prnewswire.com/news-releases/therapix-biosciences-announces-positive-data-from-recent-pre-clinical-study-for-new-drug-candidate-thx-210-300938635.html accessed 16 Sep 2021

https://www.prnewswire.com/news-releases/metagenics-releases-hemp-advantage-plus-300940215.html accessed 16 Sep 2021

Table of Abbreviations

AD	Alzheimer's disease
AEA	Anandamide or N-arachidonoylethanolamide
ALS	Amyotrophic lateral sclerosis
AN	Anorexia nervosa
ASD	Autism spectrum disorders
BCE	Before Common Era
BCP	Beta-caryophyllene
BCRP	Breast cancer resistant protein
BDNF	Brain-derived neurotrophic factor
BMI	Body Mass Index
BP	Blood pressure
CAM	Complementary and alternative medicine
CAS	Controlled Access Scheme

CBCA	Cannabichronic acid
CBD	Cannabidiol
CBDA	Cannabidiloic Acid
CBGA	Cannabigerolic acid
CBT	Cognitive Behavioural Therapy
CE	Common Era
CECD	Clinical endocannabinoid deficiency
CED	Clinical endocannabinoid deficiency (or CECD)
CNS	Central nervous system
COOH	Carboxyl Group
COPD	Chronic Obstructive Pulmonary Disease
COX	Cyclooxygenase
CSF	Cerebro spinal Fluid
CTS	Carpal tunnel syndrome
DoH	Department of Health
ECS	Endo Cannabinoid System
FAAH	Fatty acid amide hydrolase

FABP	Fatty acid binding proteins
FDA	Food and Drug Administration
GABA	Gamma amino butyric acid
GnRH	Gonadotropin-releasing hormone
Hg	Mercury
HPA	Hypothalamic-pituitary-adrenal
HPO	Hypothalamic-pituitary-ovarian
IBD	Inflammatory bowel disease
IBS	Irritable bowel syndrome
IgA	Immunoglobin A
IOP	Intra-ocular pressure
LBDDS	Lipid-based drug delivery system
LH	Luteinising hormone
MAGL	Monoacylglycerol lipase
MC	Medicinal cannabis
MoCA	Montreal Cognitive Assessment
MOE	Margin of exposure

MPTP	1-methyl-4-phenyl-1,2,3,6-tetrahyropyridine
MRSA	Methicillin-resistant Staphylococcus aureus
NAAA	N-acylethanolamine acid amide
NADA	Network of Alcohol and other Drugs Agencies
NAFLD	Non-alcoholic fatty liver disease
NGF	Nerve growth factor
NSAID	Non-steroidal anti-inflammatory drugs
OCD	Obsessive Compulsive Disorder
OEA	Oleoylethanolamide
PD	Parkinson's disease
PEA	Palmitoylethanolamide
POC	Proof-of-concept
PPAR	Peroxisome Proliferator-Activated Receptors
PTSD	Post traumatic stress disorder
RACGP	Royal Australian College of General Practitioners

SARS	Severe acute respiratory syndrome
SC	Synthetic cannabinoids
SNP	Single nucleotide polymorphisms
SSRI	Selective Serotonin Reuptake inhibitor
TCM	Traditional Chinese Medicine
TGA	Therapeutic Goods Administration
THC	Tetrahydrocannabinol
THCA	Tetrahydrocannabinolic Acid
THCV	Tetrahydrocannabivarin
TM	Trademark
TMJ	Temporomandibular Joint
TNF	Tumour necrosis factor
TRPV	Transient receptor potential cation channel subfamily V
US	Ultrasound
WADA	World Anti-Doping Agency
WM	White matter

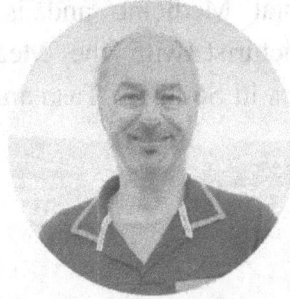

About Peter Baratosy

Peter Baratosy MB BS FACNEM is a medical doctor, lecturer, and writer on chronic diseases, especially Thyroid Disease, Gut Disorders, Hormonal Problems and Metabolic Syndrome. He has a great interest in treating chronic diseases from a more natural approach, though he does also use conventional medicines when needed. His interest in Natural Medicines led him to the study and use of medicinal cannabis in his practice which he found had a great impact on the health and well-being of his patients. Although recently retired, Dr Baratosy continues to advocate for the use of medicinal cannabis, and a more natural approach to health through his books. He graduated more than 40 years ago from the University of

Dr Peter Baratosy MB BS FACNEM

Adelaide Medical School in Australia and has over 35 years' experience as a functional medicine practitioner. He is a Fellow of the Australasian College of Nutritional and Environmental Medicine and is an accredited Medical Acupuncturist with the Medical Board of Australia. He lives in Southern Tasmania with his wife Jenny.

www.ingramcontent.com/pod-product-compliance
Lightning Source LLC
Chambersburg PA
CBHW011158220326
41597CB00028BA/4704